THE BATTLE BUDDY DIET

BY

COL (RET) ROBERT SLAY, MD, USA

First eBook Edition: February 2013

ISBN-10: 0615774113

ISBN-13: 978-0-615-774114

Table of Contents:

DEDICATION

THIS BOOK IS DEDICATED TO ALL OF MY PATIENTS, FOR THE LESSONS YOU HAVE TAUGHT ME, THE COURAGE YOU HAVE SHOWN ME, AND THE HUMILITY YOU HAVE GIVEN ME. I AM PRIVILEGED TO DO GOD'S WORK, BUT ONLY ONE PATIENT AT A TIME. THIS BOOK IS MY ATTEMPT TO REACH MORE OF YOU THAN I COULD EVER TAKE CARE OF, OR TALK TO ABOUT YOUR HEALTH. PLEASE READ IT, TAKE IT TO HEART AND STAY OUT OF THE EMERGENCY ROOM.

A SPECIAL DEDICATION GOES TO SOME BEAUTIFUL PEOPLE WHO HAVE DIED TOO SOON, FROM PREVENTABLE DISEASES. I STILL LOVE YOU ALL: MY FATHER, RD SLAY; MY BROTHER, DRAKE SLAY; JOANNE AND MONTY FISHER; AND ESPECIALLY KENNY LEVENTHAL, MY MENTOR, AND AN ANGEL IN MY LIFE.

FINALLY, I DEDICATE THIS BOOK TO MY WIFE, GAYNE BRENNEMAN, MD, "LITTLE FISH", MY "BATTLE BUDDY", FOR ALWAYS HAVING MY BACK.

COL BOB SLAY, M.D.

PREFACE:

WAGE WAR ON EXCESS WEIGHT, DISEASE AND SUFFERING, AND RECLAIM YOUR LIFE AND HEALTH.

THE "BATTLE PLAN", DETAILED IN THIS BOOK IS A SIMPLE GUIDE TO A LIFE SAVING, LIFE-STYLE CHANGE, CREATED BY A HUSBAND AND WIFE PHYSICIAN COUPLE; "BATTLE BUDDIES" WHO DID IT TOGETHER.

THE REAL TRUTH FROM TWO PHYSICIANS, MARRIED FOR 37 YEARS, WHO HAVE WON THE BATTLE AGAINST OBESITY, AND POOR NUTRITION.

LEARN HOW EXCESS BODY FAT IS A DEATH SENTENCE, WILL SHORTEN YOUR LIFE, AND LEAD TO INCESSANT SUFFERING AND DISABILITY WITH AGING.

LEARN THE TWELVE LETHAL FOODS THAT YOU SHOULD NEVER EAT AGAIN.

IF YOU HAVE HAD ENOUGH, AND WANT TO PERMANETELY ELIMINATE YOUR EXCESS BODY FAT, CHANGE WHAT YOU EAT, AND ARE WILLING ADOPT A SIMPLE, REAL LIFE-STYLE CHANGE, WITH DIET, EXERCISE AND RESISTANCE TRAINING, THIS IS HOW TO DO IT SAFELY, SURELY, AND WITH LASTING RESULTS.

LEARN HOW TO PREVENT THE OBESITY RELATED DISEASES AND CANCERS, ALL OF WHICH LEAD TO LIFE LONG DISABILITY, PAIN AND SUFFERING AND DEPENDENCY ON MEDICINES, DOCTORS AND HOSPITALS.

IDEAL BODY WEIGHT, THE RIGHT DIET AND EXERCISE WILL MAKE YOU LOOK YOUR BEST RIGHT NOW, SLOW AGING, GIVE YOU MORE ENERGY, AND RE-CHARGE YOUR SEX LIFE.

THIS IS HOW A DOCTOR COUPLE DID IT, BASED ON A CAREFUL REVIEW OF THE REAL SCIENTIFIC FACTS, GLEANED FROM CREDIBLE, WELL DONE STUDIES, CONCERNING DIET, AGING, OBESITY AND RISK FACTORS FOR MULTIPLE DISEASES.

THIS MATERIAL IS FACTUAL AND BASED ON OUR REAL LIFE EXPERIENCE. THESE ARE OUR EDUCATED OPINIONS; THE

REAL TRUTH, AS WE SEE IT, NOT INFLUENCED BY ANY AGENDA, THE FOOD INDUSTRY, OR ELIXIR SALESMEN. THIS IS WHAT WE TELL OUR FRIENDS AND FELLOW PHYSICIANS.

THIS BOOK IS A BATTLE PLAN THAT WILL LEAD YOU AND YOUR "BATTLE BUDDY" TOWARDS LIFE CHANGING VICTORY IN ONLY 4 WEEKS!

PROLOGUE:

A SIMPLE CONCEPT

We are a physician couple, husband and wife for the last 37 years. My wife's name is Gayne Brenneman, M.D., and she is a board certified cardiac anesthesiologist. My name is Robert, "Col Bob", Slay, and I am a physician, retired from the Army, board certified in Internal Medicine and Emergency Medicine.

Even though we are two well-educated doctors, it took us until our 50's to finally realize that controlling our body weight is really a life and death health issue, not a vanity issue. Despite two comprehensive medical educations, we did not realize that we fit the World Health Organization's criteria for not just "overweight" but had pushed over into "obesity" as measured by the Body Mass Index (BMI).

The BMI is only one measure of obesity based on height and weight, accepted by the scientific community as a reliable, objective measure of excessive weight. We were both had BMI's over 30, which put us into the dreaded "obese" category. The BMI has been shown to be imperfect in assessing obesity as a health risk, but it got our attention. The real culprit is abdominal or "visceral" fat, best assessed by your waist line measurement, and the ratio of your measured waist size to your hip size.

OBESITY HEALTH RISKS

We found out that being classified as having a BMI over 30, "obese", meant that we would live around 12 to 15 years less than we should, and that we would likely develop horrible chronic diseases, like diabetes, hypertension, abnormal blood lipids, atherosclerotic cardiovascular disease (ASCVD), and have a much greater chance of getting cancer. To our horror, we had blood tests for lipid profile and diabetes that were disappointing for both us. I was found to have hypertension for the first time in my life, and was diagnosed as "prediabetic", and told that I would probably need to start diabetic and hypertensive medications!

Even more convincing was the data on excessive waist circumference as a measure of obesity, which is absolutely linked to an increased risk of diabetes, hypertension, abnormal blood lipids, and CVD (metabolic syndrome) and some thirty other related diseases. Yes, male or female, if your waist circumference (measured at the belly button, without sucking in, at the widest point) is larger than your hip circumference, you are in serious trouble. If you are a male with a waist circumference of 40 inches or greater, or a female with a waist circumference of 36 inches or greater, you have a very serious health problem

Abdominal, truncal, or waist fat, is much more dangerous than fat elsewhere in the body, and has been proven to accelerate the development of multiple diseases, cancers and causes early death. My 39 inch waist (sucked in) was clearly putting me at high risk for chronic debilitating diseases and premature death.

MEDICAL LITERATURE

Rather than wade into the confusing world of diets, and weight loss magic cures, we decided to research only credible, scientifically accepted literature. We purposely did not read about any of the fad, or popular diets. We wanted to find out the facts, what really works, and how to safely lose weight and keep it off. We needed a "Battle Plan".

OPTIMAL LIFESTYLE

We wanted to lose weight without starving, while decreasing calories and maintaining a nutritious, good tasting diet that could be adapted for life. After researching all of the classic and recent studies, and all of the credible government and university based sources, concerning diet and disease, we devised a plan, our personal Battle Plan. We knew that we could not undertake the battle alone; we needed to support each other as "Battle Buddies", someone you absolutely trust, who has your back. Then in a mutually supportive effort, as "Battle Buddies", we committed to our own, (THE BATTLE BUDDY DIET) program. We pledged to try it for just 4 weeks and then reassess. We fully adapted to totally healthy diet, exercise and resistance training. The dramatic results of our 4 week effort convinced us that we should continue our new life-style for life.

We found out that we should not only avoid certain highly caloric "lethal" foods, but that what you eat really matters, not just to lose weight, but to avoid and to reverse diseases and cancers. People who resign themselves to dying of heart disease or stroke because "it runs in the family" are gravely misinformed. Only about 3 to 5% of disease is genetically inherited. The rest is brought on by the Western Diet, not exercising and other bad habits, like smoking. We were shocked to learn that a "whole foods" plant based diet, not only insures weight loss; it protects against obesity related diseases, and that this diet can, and will, even reverse them!

In just 4 weeks, supporting each other as "Battle Buddies", we both lost 8 to 10 lbs., and our waists shrunk. I was delighted to find that my blood pressure, blood lipids and diabetes screens were dramatically improving to below dangerous levels. My blood pressure came down to a very low (healthy) level. We both gained a new lease on an active, energetic life. We broke out of our unrecognized, rut, a sort of marriage depression, which I call "Middle-Aged Couple Obesity Syndrome (MACOS). We were told by friends that we looked 10 to 15 years younger. We became much more interested in each other, and realized that, "healthy is sexy". We decided to continue the battle plan and to win the war.

HOW DID YOU DO IT?

Many of our friends and coworkers wanted to know, "How did you do it?" "Why do you look so much younger, rested and full of energy?" "What do you eat, not eat, what vitamins do you take, and what kind of exercises do you do?" I started to write instructions for our friends, and my patients, but found the demand became more than I could manage. So, I decided to publish this book, and make it available to those who want to know how we, two doctors, "Battle Buddies", did it. The irony of this effort is that if this battle plan is adopted by a significant number of overweight-obese people, for even 4 weeks, the resulting weight loss, and restoration of health will probably save more lives than Gayne and I will ever "save" in our entire careers.

SIMPLE PROGRAM

THEBATTLE BUDDY DIET is a simple program that should be adopted for at least for 4 weeks. Hopefully, after seeing your own positive, dramatic results, in just 4 weeks, you will adopt this new life-style for life. It will work for anyone with a weight problem, and is especially suited for couples and families that live together, your "Battle Buddies". This program is not about vanity, it is about functional longevity. It requires only the following:

REQUIREMENTS FOR SUCCESS WITH the BATTLE BUDDY DIET

1. Not eating the "lethal food" groups.

2. Eating only healthy food.

3. Exercising/resistance training

4. Optimal sleep

What is your BMI and waist circumference? It is now or never. Declare war on obesity and reclaim your life, and sample a really healthy lifestyle. Do not surrender. The alternative is scary, relentless, and certain. Come on, you can do anything for 4 weeks. Go "all in" with your "Battle Buddy" for just 4 weeks and then see where you are. I believe you will never go back.

This book is a battle plan for your own war against excess weight, disease and suffering. It is a road map to a permanent, better, happier and healthier life. You will learn the facts, not the myths, about diet and healthy longevity. You will learn simple strategies to implement permanent changes in your diet and life-style that will profoundly change your life for the better. If you are overweight and suffering from the inevitable obesity related diseases, it is not too late. Now is the time. Commit and fight the battle, with your Battle Buddy for 4 weeks, and see what you have won. THIS MAY BE THE MOST IMPORTANT BOOK YOU EVER READ

CHAPTER 1:

WHY I WROTE THIS BOOK

We are physicians, husband and wife, both in our 60's, who finally became convinced that controlling our body weight, and what we eat, was not just a vanity issue, but was really a critical health issue; actually, a matter of life and death. We decided to research the best medical literature ourselves to find out what really works and how to safely lose weight and keep it off.

In a mutually supportive, "battle buddy" effort, we devised and committed to our own simple program of a new healthy lifestyle. In just 4 weeks, we had fully adapted to a totally healthy diet, exercise and resistance training, and in less than one year, the two of us lost all of the dangerous fat accumulated in over thirty years of marriage. We gained a new self-image, broke out of our "middle aged couple obesity syndrome" (MACOS), recovered a new sense of purpose and self-confidence. We regained a high-energy zest for life and our relationship. We became younger and healthier.

Using our own scientifically based battle plan of simple lifestyle change, we both went from overweight (BMI>25) to optimal weight in 6 months. Col. Bob went from 228 lbs. and 38" waist, to 176 lbs. and a 32" waist; Dr. Gayne from 160 lbs. and a size 14, to 128 lbs. and a size 3 to 4.

Most of our friends, fellow physicians, patients and co-workers wanted to know, "How did you do it?" "What do you eat, not eat, what vitamins do you take, what kind of exercises do you do?" There is so much conflicting information on weight control; so many temporary quick fixes, eccentric, complicated diets, magic formulas, pills and metabolic elixirs, that no one knows what really works. We made a point of not reading about any existing popular diets, so that we would not be biased in our approach.

Supported by solid scientific data, we found out what really works, what is safe, and how to keep the weight off. We also discovered that it was not just weight control and exercise that are critical, but what you eat is equally important to insure healthy functional longevity. This can only be accomplished by a sincere, commitment to real change, as detailed in this book, THE BATTLE BUDDY DIET.

The statistics on obesity and the increased risk of sudden death, stroke and heart attack are scary. Obesity is epidemic in the USA, with over 65% of the adult population either obese or overweight. Weight gain increases with age, so as our population ages, there are going to be millions of people at risk for the lethal and debilitating obesity linked diseases such as: "metabolic syndrome", hypertension, diabetes, hyperlipidemia, stroke, multiple cancers, heart attack and heart failure.

Long-term studies, involving thousands of men and women, show that obesity alone is an independent predictor premature death and cardiovascular disease. A BMI greater than 25 (overweight) puts one at risk obesity linked illnesses, as does and increased waist circumference. A man with a waist circumference greater that his hips, is 5 times more likely to die of a cardiovascular event than a man with a waist smaller than his hips. The same is true in women; those with a greater waist to hips circumference have an even higher incidence of heart attack and stroke. Heart disease is the number one killer of women in the USA, far exceeding deaths from all other causes combined. One in three women will die of a cardiovascular event.

You can assess your own risk. If you are a male and your waist is 40 inches or greater, or a female and your waist is 36 inches or greater, your prognosis is grim. Not only will you have a shortened life; it will be riddled with disease, suffering and disability.

Couples approaching middle age, fall into what I call the "Middle Age Couple Obesity" Syndrome (MACOS). They have both gained only a couple of pounds a year (one extra bagel a week will do it) over the last 15 to 20 years, and "suddenly" they are 30 to 40 lbs. overweight. They have resigned themselves to accept the fact that they are a "little heavy" and assume it is an inevitable part of normal "graceful" aging. They are sexually unappealing to each other, eat in front of the TV together, and are rapidly descending into a cascade of obesity linked illnesses. There are some 38 obesity linked illnesses and the list is growing, like: arthritis, hypertension, heart disease, sleep apnea, cancer and diabetes. Couples wonder why their lives are so unfulfilling, why they feel old, apathetic, tired, and depressed. They are where we were, in the MACOS rut.

As we lost weight, toned our bodies, ate the right foods and increased our energy level, we again became sexually attracted to each other. Others started flirting with both of us, and believe me, that had not happened for some 30 years. We decided that since other people were telling us that we "looked sexy", we should make an effort to stay healthy and "look sexy" for each other.

I wrote this book to function as your personal battle plan, a road map to permanent life-style change. This book will tell you how to lose weight, eat right, and live longer. You will learn how to always look your best and how to look sexy at any age. There are simple rules about eating, exercise and resistance training. The book tells what kind of evaluation you should have by your doctor, to assess where you are. The best battle plans are simple. This book is simple; there are no esoteric discussions of cellular physiology, just factual, practical advice and opinion, based on our comprehensive review of all of the creditable scientific literature.

With each of the diet, nutrient and exercise rules, there will be justification from medical research supporting our position. We do not pretend to be nutrition experts, and do not intend to produce a book filled with abstractions about metabolic pathways, complex recipes, calorie counting and eating schedules. This book is a battle plan for change that works, and only requires a commitment and reasonable self-discipline for 4 weeks.

The basics of nutrition physiology are simplified and explained. This book includes guidelines on blood lipid tests, hypertension evaluation, and recommended cancer screening tests for men and women. It will teach you how to really read nutrition labels, how to buy the right foods, tips on how to eat, sleep, and exercise.

We think, like us, some people, physicians, and patients who realize they are overweight, unattractive, unhealthy, at grave risk of dying prematurely, and of becoming disabled and chronically ill, will decide that they must do something about it. Such people will understand that it will take resolve, commitment and self-discipline. A short term goal of sticking to the battle plan for just 4 weeks is all that is required. In our lives of excess and instant gratification, too many of us have lost our self-discipline and personal resolve. Take it from Col. Bob, it is time to take it back, and reclaim your health. It is truly, now or never!

We are two board-certified physicians, husband and wife, who studied all of the best, credible scientific sources related to obesity, losing weight, health risks, diets, nutrients, vitamins, supplements and strategies for staying healthy and looking your best. We have produced a battle plan of potentially life-saving, life-style guidelines, facts and rules. We wrote the book for our friends and patients, so they could get healthier, too. This book is especially for our fellow physicians, since they must "walk the walk" to "talk the talk". This program will work for anyone, at any age, and will change the lives and relationships of those who commit to this plan. Give it just 4 weeks and you will never want to go back to the "Dark Side".

CHAPTER 2:

COL BOB'S STORY

I was an athlete in high school and college, and always considered myself somewhat of a stud. Of course, that was when I weighed 169 lbs. at 5' 9" tall, had a six-pack and a 32" waist. I graduated from the Virginia Military Institute and went through Medical School on an Army scholarship. I completed training in internal medicine and became board certified in internal medicine. I became a career Army physician.

I practiced Internal Medicine for only one year, and then realized that I was stuck in a small office most of the time, seeing hoards of self-destructive, noncompliant, patients with self-induced chronic diseases, like emphysema, diabetes, heart disease, high blood pressure, and hyperlipidemia in mostly obese patients. Despite my heroic efforts to get them to change, or even just to take their medications, almost all of them went on to continue their self-destructive life-styles, and kept smoking, eating the wrong foods, gaining weight and getting sicker.

Eventually, after miserable lives of debility and dependency, cancer or the nasty cardiovascular diseases like heart attack, congestive heart failure, renal failure, stroke, and atherosclerosis would take them out. I felt that I was "pissing in the wind", seeing one patient every 9 minutes, all with variations of the same diseases, all relentlessly spiraling down the drain. I decided to change specialties. Office medicine was just too boring, gave me no feeling of accomplishment, and besides, you had to write all of those redundant prescriptions. I always felt pushing medicines never really addressed the primary problem: most of these diseases were self-induced. Why didn't someone tell these patients that losing weight and eating healthy foods could have prevented their diseases, or even reversed them? No one told them, even me, because I didn't know.

As more of an action oriented physician, I gravitated towards Emergency Medicine. It is medicine, just the way I like it. It is a medical practice with a great eclectic variety of challenging illness and trauma, with a chance to intervene in life and death situations and to truly make a difference. The emergency department is blessed with variety, for better or worse. You have to know a great deal about all of the other subspecialties, since virtually any homosapien, with any medical problem, presenting to an emergency room anywhere in the US is entitled to complete care. I think of my practice as operating in a high risk Trailways station of medicine.

The real-life struggles of the patients and their families, the vignettes, the joy and the sorrow, and the chance to emergently intervene, provided me a palpable sense of accomplishment, and made the work fun. I began work in a large Army emergency department, started the first Emergency Medicine training program in the military and became board certified in Internal Medicine and Emergency Medicine.

In those early days, my serum testosterone level frequently exceeded my IQ, and clouded my judgment; so when invited, I joined the super-secret, anti-terrorist Delta Force. The members of Delta are "the elite" of the SEALS, Special Forces, and the Army Rangers. Needless to say, since your life depended on being in shape, we spent a great deal of duty time conditioning, lifting weights and training. It was fairly easy to stay in shape with mandatory two time a day workouts, 6 days a week, weather you felt like it or not. There were Army regulations that restricted weight for active duty soldiers, and could be used to force retirement or separation of the "fighting fatties". Obese soldiers just do not inspire the confidence of the public and make larger, sweaty, slower targets for the enemy.

My insidious creep towards obesity began after I retired from the Army at the age of 41. I had no more Army fat regulations to meet and no enforced workouts. I was also a new father of two young children. In retrospect, the kids are one of the major reasons that I got fat. With my odd hours of work, and Gayne's demanding medical training, we barely had time to work and then to drive the kids to all of their soccer, scouts, music lessons, ballet, other teams, and the unending school events. Does any of this sound familiar?

Any plans for an evening at home were frequently disrupted by those unplanned, desperation, trips to the all-night Target to pick up the poster board required for the school project due in the morning. It became harder and harder to schedule my work outs or even to make a healthy dinner. We were both totally exhausted. We ate carry-out fast food, or microwaved some processed food and ate expedient, very unhealthy meals.

Worse still, was the fact that our kids wore us down, and before we knew it, we were allowing trips to the fast food joints, ordering home delivery mega pizza (it's ok, the "Hawaiian" is less caloric and healthier, we told ourselves!), We began eating chips in front of the TV, cooking big steaks on the grill, and even sneaking the kids' Snickers bars. If you have kids, you know how that happens.

When I relented and stopped at the fast-food places with the kids, after they had worn me down, with their incessant James Brown mantra, "Please, please, please, please." I would always order only a diet coke for myself, because, "I didn't eat fast food." Of course, as the kids came to expect, I would always "just taste" a few (or more) of their fries. "Get your own, Dad, you always eat ours". Of course, that was not true, because I didn't eat fast food.

I hardly noticed that I had to buy larger and larger pants, and even shirts. Since mens' pants tend to increase in 2" increments, going from a 32" waist to a 34", really meant that my waist was a only 33", but I always got them a little larger because they "might shrink". And boy, did they shrink! So much so, that I had to move up to 36". But it would only be for a while. I knew that I could lose the weight any time I decided to, and would "eventually".

It became even worse working in the ER, since I wore scrub pants at work. The scrub pants draw strings are color coded by size of the scrubs. I transitioned through the orange (small), green (medium), black (large), and finally graduated to the dreaded red (extra-large) drawstrings. In the locker room with the other expanding doctors, putting on our scrubs, we all complained that "they are making these scrubs smaller and smaller". I agreed, "Yeah they are using less material to make them, to save money!" I thought I must be going color blind.

Finally, I had to buy 38" pants, but only because I was really a 37" waist and the pants will shrink...and so on. The thought that I might actually be getting heavier, never registered with me. I was just getting older, and a little weight gain was part of that process. I did not want to be weighed, because our obviously inaccurate home scale showed that I had topped 228 lbs., and that was impossible!

Initially driven by vanity, I made heroic efforts to lose the weight. I would buy only low-fat or no-fat products, but that did not help. Why? I call it the "coffee shop conspiracy". While getting my coffee shop coffee, to my absolute delight, I discovered that they had "low-fat" muffins, "low-fat" bagels and even "low-fat" cream cheese to put on them. Of course, the 250 to 300 calories per low-fat item and the excessive grams of sugar and carbohydrates was not mentioned. The more I looked, the more such products seemed available. I ate only "no fat", "reduced fat", and "lite" food products exclusively, and got even fatter.

One extra bagel a week, an extra 250 calories, translates to almost 4 lbs. gained a year, or 40 lbs. in just ten years. So I fought it by exercising more, trying a variety of diets, liquid, fruit, protein, food plans, and even fasting. I would lose 5 or 10 lbs. in a few weeks, but felt like a returning POW. So, as in every diet of this type, I regained the weight and became a fat guy who had exercised himself into great shape.

While pulling on my X-Large scrub pants with the red draw strings, I was horrified by the image of the red string looking like a tether from the Hindenburg, obscured by my 6 month pregnant-looking belly hanging over the scrub pants. Nurses, and other people at work, would tell me, "You don't look fat. You look good for your age". Other people around me seemed fatter than me, and besides you are expected to be heavier when you get older. Isn't that part of "graceful aging"? Look at Dr. Weil, all tubby and graceful. I thought that's how aging is meant to be.

Like all fat guys in denial, I would suck in my stomach, flex up my arms, hold my breath and peer into the waist-high bathroom mirror each morning and conclude, "I don't look so fat, and I'm in better shape than other guys my age". I found that without my glasses, if I kind of squinted my eyes, while fiercely sucking in my stomach, looking into a foggy mirror, I could almost see the long-lost 6 pack under the fat. I looked "pretty good", certainly not obese.

My moment of clarity came at the age of 55, when I weighed 228 lbs., with a 38" plus, waist and a BMI of 35 (obese). There it was, on the internet, the dreaded word. The World Health Organization (WHO) had officially classified me as "obese". Our vacation pictures from that summer, made me look particularly fat, since many were snapped using digital technology, quicker than I could suck in my stomach. Even with my stomach sucked in, the guy I saw in those pictures looked like a middle aged, round-faced, generously jouled, fat guy. That is not how I look! That guy in the pictures was really not me. The fat guy in the pictures was the person I had become, not the person I really was.

At that same time, Gayne had a similar revelation by calculating her own BMI (obese, too) and critically appraising her own vacation pictures showing a bloated, broad-hipped, flabby-armed, middle-aged, fat mom. Even worse, our yearly blood work, the lipid profiles, and diabetic screens, showed bad numbers; mine worse than hers.

I was further shocked to find out that for the first time, I was having blood pressures that were borderline high and might have to be treated. Finally, my internist and I were unpleasantly surprised to find that my fasting blood sugar was a "little on the high side". Oh My God, I was beginning to develop the metabolic syndrome; hypertension, abnormal blood fats, and insulin resistance, or the beginning of diabetes. That couldn't be a good thing. But I was in great shape, and gracefully aging, there must be some mistake.

We were both profoundly depressed. Our relationship was strained by the fact that we had almost no sex-life. I thought it was because fat people like me, and like Gayne, were not sexy or that you just normally decreased sex in marriages longer than 20 years. Our mutual lack of a positive self-image destroyed our individual sexual self-esteem and further stressed our relationship.

Frustrated, we found ourselves commenting on what the other was eating, or on how good they "used to look". It got so bad, that I finally broke down and told her, truthfully, that "yes", those pants she just pulled on, really were "a little too tight". That comment did not improve our sex life.

Then came the coup de gras, and our ultimate salvation: the discovery that excessive body fat not only makes you look and feel terrible, it is deadly. For the first time there was a compelling reason to lose the weight. We did a comprehensive review of the very best medical literature on obesity, to find out how to really lose weight and keep it off. We knew that fad diets would not work or be sustainable. Rather, we went to the best nutrition sources in the world; such as the NIH, WHO, university medical center web sites, and peer reviewed quality medical studies, in order to draw our own conclusions.

We came up with our own simple battle plan that we knew would require, acceptance, commitment and discipline. We decided to mutually commit and go "all in" for one month. We did not want a rigid diet that required exact measuring of servings, counting points, or doing complicated food exchanges. It had to be a program that told us what you should and should not eat, ways to avoid eating the wrong things, and recommendations for the nutrients that may have real scientifically proven benefit.

The keystone of this battle plan was not just diet, but the absolute necessity of regular exercise and resistance training.

After just 4 weeks of adopting our plan, I lost 10 lbs., and felt a new energy and hope. I had grieved for some of the lethal foods I had to forgo, but I had started to really like the new whole foods diet. I was never hungry and continued to exercise. Because of our immediate 4 week results, we decided to continue the battle plan another month. My Battle Buddy, Gayne, had my back, and vice versa, supporting each other in sticking to the battle plan.

Weeks turned to months, and after eight months I weighed 176 lbs. (loss of >50 lbs.), had a waist of 32" and a healthy BMI of 25. Gayne has had similar spectacular results. We both have normal lipid numbers and I have normal blood pressure. We have more energy, are not depressed and have a recharged sex life. We tell each other that we look good, because we do. Our relationship has been resuscitated and we feel that we are "in love" again. Most importantly, we know that we stand a good chance of living around 12 or 15 years longer than we would have, while remaining healthy, self-sufficient, mobile and optimistic.

Our overweight friends and co-workers tell us we are getting "too skinny", that we don't need to lose any more weight. That's true, all we have to do is maintain the current weight, and that is easy with our "Do eat" and "Do not eat" foods and eating tips. People now think that we are both 10 to 12 years younger than we are, because as you will see, the key to looking younger and functioning younger is achieving your optimal body weight and eating the right foods.

Our friends, family and patients want to know how we did it. That is why I wrote this book. Just as we would tell a best friend, this is how we, a two doctor couple, permanently changed our life style, lost the weight together and re-vitalized our relationship. This is how we did it. Just the facts as we found them. We expect controversy, and do not pretend to be experts on nutrition. We just know that this battle plan is supported by creditable medical research, is safe and it works. There is no downside or risk to this battle plan.

Finally, I decided that my corpulent cohorts, the pudgy doctors, struggling to get into their shrinking scrubs every day, could use a little help, too. Most physicians know nothing about diet, nutrition or healthy life-style. They see obese patients by the score, ravaged by obesity linked diseases and cancers. How can they realistically tell their patients to adopt a healthy life style if they do not do it themselves? It has been shown that it is very unlikely that an overweight physician will counsel an overweight patient on diet or life style. It would be like me telling the patient not to smoke with a package of Marlboros in my scrubs top pocket.

Imagine that you have had an obese doctor for years that you came to see for appointments on a regular basis, to address the mounting problems with your obesity and related maladies. After a period of time, he suddenly started to look like Paul Ryan, seemed more energetic, optimistic and appeared to be 10 years younger. You might ask how he did it, and now he might even be willing to discuss it with you.

Physician, heal thyself! Thus, this book, <u>THE BATTLE BUDDY DIET</u>, is an attempt to get the word out, not just to patients, but to physicians, so that they will apply this diet and life style to themselves. Just as the Surgeon General came down on smoking in the 1960's, with the scientific evidence that it caused cancer and disease, I hope to sound the alarm about obesity related diseases. Before the smoking revelations of the 1960's, almost 50% of physicians smoked, now it is fewer than 5%. Hopefully this message will help do the same for the 60% of physicians that are overweight or obese.

CHAPTER 3:

WHY ARE WE FAT?

OVER EATING/EATING THE WRONG FOODS/NOT EXERCISING

Why are we made to feel guilty about the fact that the fat person squeezed into the plane seat next to us does not have enough room? I suppose it is because we have been told that obesity is a disease, and we feel that overweight people are "infected", through no fault of their own. That is usually not the case. The fact is that even though there are genetic, hormonal, and endocrine causes of obesity, 95% is caused by over eating, eating the wrong foods, and not exercising. It is simple, more calories are taken in than are being burned for energy, those that are not burned are stored as fat.

Of course there are lots of reasons for over eating, including; eating disorders, like binge eating and a myriad of psychological problems, most often depression. Environmental factors are a major factor in the current world-wide obesity pandemic. Study after study, here and in developing countries, have shown that the conversion to the Western Diet (mammalian meat, processed meats, refined grains, processed foods, sweets and deserts, fried foods, and dairy products) will dramatically increase obesity in a previously normal weight population. In so doing, obesity linked diseases will increase, most importantly cancers and metabolic syndrome, the gateway to atherosclerotic cardiovascular disease (ASCVD), diabetes and hypertension.

We have been duped by the food industry, who push really unhealthy, "great tasting" food in massive quantities. We have been victimized by "low fat" and "lite" products, like muffins, not taking into account the carbohydrates, sugars and calories. Many of the fats used in cooking and preparation of processed foods have been shown to increase the amount of bad lipids and triglycerides in our blood, and to stimulate intravascular inflammation and coagulation, the harbingers of heart attacks and stroke.

The Trans-fatty acids are very dangerous and found in the majority of processed foods. They are man-made fatty acids, created by altering the molecular structure of natural fats, by heating and "hydrogenating" vegetable oils to make them solid at room temperature. Such Trans-fats do not exist in nature, but are in abundance in processed foods, and deep fried foods. Recent studies have shown them to be truly lethal substances, because they increase bad fats, lower good fats, and increase atherosclerosis progression by increasing systemic inflammation. They are highly caloric and make you fat.

The number of unhealthy calories that can be consumed quickly is prodigious. A woman with a 1,800 calorie daily requirement will have taken in 83% of her total daily caloric requirement (1,500 calories) by eating one fast food burger, a small order of fries, and a small soft drink. It is horrifying to learn that eating one, single potato chip (14 calories) a day, over your daily caloric requirements, would add enough calories to cause around a 1 ½ pound weight gain a year!

Fewer than 14% of Americans exercise on a regular basis. We seem to walk as little as possible. We like to eat large servings of fatty fried chips, and a staggering variety of processed foods while watching television. We love fatty snacks, candy and soft drinks especially while traveling in the car. We love buttered popcorn in the movies. I loved ice cream in the middle of the night.

Overweight and obesity related illness now top smoking for medical costs in the U.S. Experts see the current epidemic of obesity as the illness that is already beginning to overwhelm the health care system, as the Baby Boomers age, and get fatter and as their obese children develop illnesses like diabetes.

Since 1991 until 2000, obesity in the U.S. rose 60%. Currently, almost 70% of all American adults are overweight. Obesity has the same impact on health as aging 20 years in adults. We learned in medical school to use the 70 kg. (154 pounds) man as average size, but a 2006 study published by JAMA, showed the average weight of a man to be 88 kg. (195 lbs.) and the average weight of a female to be 75kg. (165 lbs.). I can only guess it has gone up since then.

Even more alarming is the waist circumference data on men and women. Abdominal or central obesity is most commonly assessed by measuring waist circumference or waist-to-hip ratio. From 1988-1994 to 1999-2000, mean waist circumference of adult Americans increased from 43.3 in. to 44.8 in. in men and from 40.3 in. to 41.9 in. in women. Surely it has increased even more since then. In general, the hip to waist ratio is a better measure of dangerous obesity than the BMI. If your waist is larger than your hips, male or female, you are at significant risk for all of the obesity linked diseases and cancers. All of these, people with their waist larger than their hips, have a "terminal illness" that will relentlessly progress, bring them unimaginable suffering and will kill them prematurely.

The bottom line is that we have a country full of fat, sick people. I am shocked by the terrifying accelerating obesity in children and adolescents in the USA. Parents seem unaware of the permanent harm they are doing to their children by allowing them to eat all of the wrong foods, not to exercise, and allowing them to live an unhealthy life-style.

We have found with our own two children, setting the example is the best policy. Teenagers and college students can get junk food 24 hours a day despite your best efforts. There is hope; several studies support the fact that eventually most children will ultimately adopt a diet and life style similar to that of their parents.

There is no easy or magic way to lose weight and keep it off. Never in the history of the published medical literature has a quick-fix, gimmick diet worked to take weight off and keep it off for 5 years. All of the myths about fruit juices burning more calories, or the benefits of an all-protein diet, all egg-diet, all meat diet, green coffee beans, raspberry extract, ad nausem: do not work in the long run. Some stimulants, and energy drinks can increase metabolism and decrease appetite, but have a high downside risk for potentially increasing blood pressure, the risk of stroke, heat injury, and cardiac arrhythmia.

Please do not waste your money on special "fat absorbers", "metabolic boosters", or other pills and elixirs that "burn fat" while allowing you eat anything you want, or worse, even claim to cause "weight loss while you sleep". Miracle elixirs are as old as recorded history. They didn't work then and they don't work now. Some of the organized weight loss programs, or healthy food delivery programs can promote weight loss in the short run, but it cannot be sustained without a comprehensive sustained lifestyle change.

The answer is simple. You must adapt a new lifestyle. Stick to your battle plan. You must change what you eat permanently. You must exercise every single day and do resistance exercises 3 times a week. Any questions?

CHAPTER 4:

EXCESS BODY FAT: A DEATH SENTENCE

BODY MASS INDEX (BMI)

What is your BMI? There is a 65% chance that it is greater than 25, meaning that you are either overweight (25-30), obese (30-35), morbidly obese (35-40) or super obese (40-45). In Asian populations, the WHO now suggests a lower BMI as being overweight (23 or greater), because of their tendency to develop truncal obesity but have thin, light limbs.

BMI can be calculated by dividing your weight in pounds by your height in inches squared x 703. An alternative calculation is: multiple your weight in pounds x 703, then divide that answer by your height in inches, then divide that answer by your height in inches again. There are multiple BMI calculators on line that can give you a quick answer. Be honest about your real measured height and weight!

If you have a BMI greater than 25, then you are overweight. I know this is a shock, because you do not believe you are overweight, or think it is not a health problem, just an aesthetic problem. I know, you have "big bones", "lots of muscle", "retain fluid", a "thyroid problem" or have "slow metabolism". No, you are still overweight. The higher the BMI, the greater chance you will die much sooner than your thinner friends and you will most likely become a sick invalid in the remaining years of your life.

It is possible to have a high BMI and not be at risk for metabolic syndrome, if you are a woman and have only subcutaneous fat; and a "pear" rather than an "apple" shape. That means women with a waist smaller than their hips, even obese. In fact, that body habitus has been shown to protect against heart disease and stroke (CVD). Subcutaneous fat, in women, with a waist smaller than their hips, may have a role in decreasing vascular inflammation. I wish we knew why.

WAIST, ABDOMINAL, OBESITY

It's not just the BMI; the distribution of the fat is critical. Waist circumference (measured around the belly button, without "sucking it in") is an absolute predictor of the metabolic syndrome. You are in trouble if your waist circumference is greater than your hips, male or female.

METABOLIC SYNDROME

Metabolic syndrome is a constellation of linked diseases: hypertension, insulin resistance, diabetes type II, low good cholesterol (HDL), high bad cholesterol (LDL) and high triglycerides. This condition accelerates atherosclerosis, aging, stroke, diabetes, vascular insufficiency, infections, heart attack, heart failure, cancers and sudden premature death.

The abdominal fat, both lining the inside of the abdominal wall, and stored around and in intrabdominal organs, like the liver, intestines, pancreas, and even the heart, is different from subcutaneous fat. It secretes a staggering number of enzymes, vasoactive substances, cytokines (inflammatory substances), hormones (?), and a tissue necrosis (tissue breakdown) factor that has been shown to directly inflame the lining of arteries, accelerating unstable plaque formation, and ASCVD.

Overweight people that develop metabolic syndrome will live some 15 to 20 years less than their disease free cohorts. That means they will be dying around their late 50's to early 60's. Not only will they die sooner, they will be chronically ill getting there. As they develop the associated diseases, they will become totally dependent on immediately accessible medical care, never ending appointments, blood tests, and expensive medications critical to just staying alive. They lose mobility, function, and independence, and usually ending up as complete bed-ridden invalids.

WOMEN: GREATER THREAT OF ASCVD

Women are at high risk for obesity related illnesses, especially metabolic syndrome and ASCVD. Heart disease is the number one killer of women in the U.S., with the total deaths far exceeding the sum of all of the female cancers (breast, ovary, cervix) combined, each year. Women stand a 1 in 3 chance of dying of ASCVD (heart attack, heart failure, or stroke). They have more heart attacks than men do much worse than men after a heart attack. If women survive a heart attack, they almost always develop heart failure, an absolute death sentence.

AFRICAN AMERICAN, HISPANIC WOMEN

African American women are particularly at risk, with 15 to 20% being morbidly obese, with a BMI greater than 40. Around 80% of African-American women over the age of 40 are overweight or obese. Hispanic women are becoming obese at the greatest rate, and are experiencing an epidemic of metabolic syndrome at a younger and younger age.

OBESITY IS NOT A VANITY ISSUE

Obesity is not an aesthetic issue; it is a matter of life and death. If I told you that you have cancer and a limited life expectancy and can expect suffering, you would be shocked. Overweight and obesity related illness kill some 300,000 people a year, second only to tobacco related diseases that account for 500,000 deaths a year. Given the current trends in epidemic obesity occurring in aging Baby Boomers, children and adolescents, obesity related deaths will surpass tobacco related deaths within the next 3 years.

It is sobering to realize that people do not view excessive weight as a health problem, just an appearance problem. Many are more concerned about their thinning hair, getting a pedicure, or contracting brain cancer from cell phones. Most people attempt to lose weight only to improve their appearance, and are always looking for easy ways to lose the weight without changing their life-style. When "diets" work, such weight losses are always temporary, discourage further dieting, and have never been shown to stop continuing weight gain or the associated diseases.

AVOID THE DRAIN

I picture all of us floating in the "pond of life". The pond has a drain, and eventually we will all go down that drain. We would all like to peacefully float far away from the drain as long as possible, then when the time comes, to quietly drift down the drain (die in your sleep). Those who are overweight drift towards the drain quicker and soon find themselves caught up in the chaos of the drain whirlpool, where they will circle the drain, suffering, in pain every waking moment, struggling just to keep their heads above the water, in a vortex of debilitating diseases, just trying just to stay alive and then finally being mercifully sucked down.

The trick to staying away from the drain is to reduce or eliminate your chance of getting obesity related diseases, especially metabolic syndrome. Multiple studies of thousands of men and women followed for 30 to 50 years, all show that eating a whole food diet low in processed foods, animal fat, sugars, and dairy fat, combined with ideal body weight, exercise and resistance training, almost guarantees disease free functional longevity. It is the only way to peacefully float away from the drain.

IT IS THE LIFE-STYLE

When early studies showed significant decrease in obesity linked diseases in people eating a whole foods, prudent diet (high in whole foods, grains, vegetables, and fish), investigators had concerns that it might not just be the diet, because people who ate such a diet "were more likely to be active, and exercise". No kidding! We were later to discover that exercise, ideal body weight, and even weight training (a healthy life-style) are common in this group, and they were far more likely to be active, independent, pain free, mentally alert and happy.

Life-style, plain and simple, is the major difference in older people who stay functional, independent and live the longest life, free of debilitating disease. They are proof that a prudent diet, ideal weight, exercise and even weight training, can extend life and are critical to avoiding a multitude of painful, diseases and cancers.

COMMIT TO 30 DAYS

If think you and your Battle Buddy cannot tolerate such a drastic change in life-style, please try it for only 30 days. If you really commit, stick to it, and are honest with yourself, your results will pleasantly shock you; you will see and feel a difference. Then you may decide, as we did, that this diet is acceptable for another month; it tastes good, is plenty of food, adds nutrients, cuts down inflammation, aids weight loss and weight maintenance, and yields more energy and a new enthusiasm for life and your relationships.

Though we expect criticism from the "experts" on THE BATTLE BUDDY DIET program, it is hard to understand how a diet high in whole grains and vegetables, and including plant protein, fish, non-fat dairy, and fruits can be harmful. Likewise, we believe striving for your ideal body weight is not a vanity issue: if you are overweight, it is your most serious health risk and is much more likely to kill you than using your cell phone or standing to close to the microwave. Finally, incorporating regular exercise and resistance training can only be a good thing, and in fact, it has been shown to help maintain weight, decrease truncal or waist fat, decrease the incidence of diabetes, ASCVD, dementia and stroke.

EVEN A 10% WEIGHT LOSS CAN SAVE YOUR LIFE

If you enter into this program and fall short of ideal BMI, you still will add quality years to your life even if you lose only 10% of your body weight. Even in patients with truncal obesity, a 10% weight loss, paired with exercise, has been shown to reduce the fat from the waist preferentially, and has significantly delayed or prevented metabolic syndrome in obese patients.

CHAPTER 5:

EXCESSIVE BODY FAT AND INFLAMMATION

INFLAMMATION: THE REAL PROBLEM

Body fat, measured by the BMI and waist circumference, is central to the real causes of acquired diabetes II, atherosclerosis, abnormal blood lipids, multiple cancers and cardiovascular diseases, like hypertension, stroke, and heart attack. There is exciting new data that supports the theory that the abdominal fat cells, (truncal obesity), are a major cause of chronic inflammation in the vascular system.

Inflammation is now accepted as the major cause of the vascular changes of atherosclerosis. A finding of systemic inflammation, as indicated by a single, inexpensive blood test, the C-reactive protein (CRP) has been shown to absolutely predict the risk of ASCVD in women with a "high" level of CRP who had "normal" serum lipids (lipid profile), and no other risk factors for ASCVD. The same data is emerging in long-term studies of men.

C-REACTIVE PROTEIN

The CRP is a serum marker, a protein substance produced by the liver, in response to chronic inflammation in the body. For example, chronic rheumatoid arthritis patients typically have a high CRP. There is growing evidence that inflammation (maybe CRP itself) initiates the beginning of the atherosclerosis plaque formation in arterial vessels, with the recruitment of destructive cells, white blood cells, moncytes, and even the CRP itself, being incorporated into the plaque. Incidentally, chronic rheumatoid patients, lupus patients and patients with ulcerative colitis, all chronic inflammatory diseases with high CRP levels, have been shown to be 70% more likely to have a cardiac event and 50% more likely to have potentially lethal emboli from blood clots in the vascular system than patients without those diseases.

Chronic periodontal disease is a chronic inflammatory disease, which affects over half of Americans over 30 years old that has been proven to cause an increased risk of pancreatic cancer. I can only guess that Steve Jobs, in his early non-bathing, working around the clock years, when he admitted neglecting his health, might have neglected his teeth, and might have had periodontal disease that led to his pancreatic cancer.

Periodontal disease is a chronic low grade infection of the gums and teeth. It has been shown to increase the incidence of certain head and neck cancers, melanoma, lung, bladder and prostate cancers in men. Full blown periodontitis, involving the gums, periodontal ligament, and bone supporting the teeth is a systemic inflammatory disease. It increases the serum inflammatory markers, including CRP, and in so doing, causes a greater risk of ASCVD, diabetes, hypertension, and stroke. Periodontitis has not been proven the cause of these diseases, but is strongly linked as a risk factor for developing them. Bottom line: eliminate it from your life by flossing, brushing and getting regular teeth cleaning.

Several credible studies have found a strong correlation between inflammatory markers in the blood and "old age" frailty. Older patients with greater inflammation as measured by the CRP, and other markers of in the blood, were heavier than those without inflammatory changes, especially those with truncal obesity. They were much less able to function independently and died about 8 years sooner than their healthier cohorts.

In 1982, two forward thinking gastroenterologists committed heresy in the world of medical science by suggesting that perhaps peptic ulcer disease could be secondary to an inflammatory response in the stomach caused by a bacterial infection. Everyone in medicine knew that ulcers were caused by stress, eating spicy foods and excessive stomach acid. Of course, this bacterial infection theory was uniformly rejected by their colleagues, and their data were not taken seriously when presented at international medical meetings. By now you know that this theory went on to be proven and now allows definitive, curative treatment of a significant number of ulcer victims. Likewise, it has become apparent that ASCVD is accelerated by chronic inflammation, not just due to cholesterol building up in the arteries like scale in an old pipe.

Cardiovascular researchers are showing a greater correlation with arterial vascular inflammation and the development of atherosclerosis. It seems that when inflammation increases, so do the bad lipids, and the triglycerides and good lipids decrease. Perhaps all these years of treating the high lipids with the statin drugs has really only been decreasing inflammation (they do). That might also explain the fact that male patients maintained on low dose aspirin live longer and have fewer cardiovascular events than those that do not take aspirin. Though low dose aspirin reduces the tendency of blood to clot, it reduces inflammation and in so doing, reduces the progression of ASCVD, and even decreases the incidence of some types of obesity related malignancies (colon).

So how do fat cells cause inflammation? The problem starts with the adipocyte or fat cell. There is still controversy regarding whether or not fat cells can divide or grow in number after birth. We are born with millions of them anyway, and they are capable of growing much larger when loaded with stored fat. They are all over the body, but are concentrated around the waist, hips, and buttocks depending on our genetic pre-disposition, sex and race. When I am suturing lacerations in the ER, the patients are always shocked to see subcutaneous fat protruding from their cut finger.

Fat cells coat your entire body like a tight fitting body suit, just under your skin. That is one reason that weight gain can be so insidious; in the beginning you just kind of get thicker all over. At the same time, other fat cells in your intestines, liver, heart and everywhere else, start to increase in size, swollen with stored fat. That why your abdomen begins to look 6 months pregnant as you become obese. It is coated with a thick layer of fat just under the skin, but is protruding because your intestines and internal organs are coated by, and filled with fat and need more room. This waist fat, or truncal/intestinal/abdominal fat, is particularly dangerous and is an independent risk factor for premature death, ASCVD, stroke and diabetes.

INFLAMMATORY SUBSTANCES FROM FAT CELLS

To incorporate all of this increasing fat storage, the fat cells become metabolically active. To process and store the fat, the cells must release enzymes, and other powerful compounds that cause systemic effects. One of the active group of proteins released are the cytokines. The cytokines are used to help break down fat, but are known to cause intravascular inflammation. In fact, lipid cytokine levels directly correlate with the amount of body fat, especially truncal obesity, and decrease dramatically with weight loss, even with as little as 10% weight loss, especially when lost from the waist.

In multiple other studies, levels of measured CRP showed the same relationship: more truncal body fat means higher levels. Losing truncal body fat markedly decreases CRP levels. Not all patients with a high CRP are obese, but the vast majority of patients with truncal obesity and early stages of atherosclerosis, have high CRP levels.

Chronic infection is being looked for as a cause for elevated levels of CRP in patients with ASCVD. There have been some studies showing that certain types of infections, like chronic viral disease, chlamydia or other bacterial infections have been linked to increased inflammation and higher CRP levels. There are multiple reasons for the development of ASCVD, but a strong, independent predictor of patients at significant risk for progressive, lethal consequences of ASCVD is available with the CRP test.

FATTY MEALS AND TRANS-FATS: INCREASE INFLAMMATION

There is strong evidence that high fat meals, or processed foods with Trans-fats, cause an immediate reaction within the arterial vascular system, increasing resistance to blood flow, increasing the stiffness of arteries, and directly causing intravascular inflammation within minutes of eating such a meal. The number harmful intravascular free radicals immediately increase, further increasing vascular inflammation.

There is evidence that the man-made Trans-fats are directly incorporated into the lining of the arteries causing the body's immune system to attack them as foreign. Not only does this create more inflammation, it leads to a buildup of cellular debris in the vessel wall, called plaque, the sine qua non of ASCVD. Continued intra vascular inflammation, creates a mature unstable plaque (think of a pimple ready to "pop") inside of the arterial wall, or endothelium, which then ruptures into the artery releasing intensely inflammatory substances. This released inflammatory cellular debris then causes a blood clot, blocking the artery and causing ischemia, or lack of cellular oxygen to the muscle. If that vessel is a coronary artery and the muscle is the heart, it is called a myocardial infarction or heart attack. Over half the time, the first symptom of a heart attack is sudden death.

HOW TO DECREASE INFLAMMATION

Thousands of men and women on whole food, prudent, non-Western diets, have very low systemic measures of inflammation, and tend to live much longer, with significantly lower incidents of ASCVD, stoke, abnormal lipids, cancers and diabetes. It has recently been demonstrated that giving a select number of patients with high CRP levels and abnormal lipids, a prudent whole food diet, high in grains, vegetables and low in fats, was as good as statin medications in improving lipids and decreasing inflammation. Such diets are referred to as "anti-inflammatory" diets. This prudent diet group, had the additional benefit of losing weight and improving their blood pressure, and has certainly increased their odds of living longer and healthier lives.

BLOOD TEST

The best blood test for systemic inflammation is the high-sensitivity CRP, or the (hs-CRP). It has emerged as the most cost effective inflammatory serum marker to assess cardiovascular risk. It is widely available, and costs approximately $30; significantly cheaper than the usual lipid profile. I strongly feel that this test should be a part of screening all patients for ASCVD. Insist on it. If your physician will not run the test, or does not know about CRP and risk of ASCVD, get a new physician.

THE BATTLE BUDDY DIET program attacks systemic inflammation with diet and lifestyle.

CHAPTER 6:

DISEASES DIRECTLY LINKED TO OBESITY

CARDIOVASCULAR: hypertension, coronary artery disease, cardiomyopathy, heart failure, accelerated atherosclerosis, pulmonary hypertension, left ventricular hypertrophy, cor pulmonale, blood clots in the legs, blood clots to the lungs.

CENTRAL NERVOUS: stroke (ischemic and hemorrhagic), parathesias, carpal tunnel syndrome, idiopathic intracranial hypertension, premature dementia, neuralgia paresthetica.

GASTROINTESTINAL: Gall bladder diseases, nonalcoholic hepatitis, fatty liver, gastric acid reflux, reflux esophagitis.

RESPIRATORY: obstructive sleep apnea, hypoventilation syndrome, respiratory infections, asthma.

PSYCHOLOGICAL: depression, eating disorders, low self-esteem, marital problems, social stigmatization.

MUSCULOSKELETAL: accelerated osteoarthritis, slipped hip, back disease (disc, fractures), sciatica, Coxa vara, slipped capital femoral epiphyses (hip),Blount's disease (abnormality of lower leg, tibia), Legg-Calve-Perthes disease (avascular necrosis of the femoral head, hip joint), lumbago (chronic back pain).

METABOLIC: insulin resistance, hyperinsulinemia, diabetes II, high bad lipids (LDL), low good lipids (HDL) and high triglycerides.

REPRODUCTIVE: anovulation, premature puberty (starts when girls reach 98 pounds), infertility, polycystic ovaries, decreased levels of testosterone, diminished sex drive, hypogonadism, sub-fecundity, stress incontinence and probably erectile dysfunction.

OBSTETRIC AND PERINATAL: hypertension of pregnancy, large babies, pelvic dystocia (too small for baby).

SKIN: Intertrigo (infections), edema or swelling of the lower legs, venous varicosities, chronic stasis leg ulcers, fibromyalgia, acanthosis nigricans (darkened skin), hirsuitism, cellulitis, carbuncle, cutaneous abscess.

CANCERS: breast, colon, prostate, uterine, gall bladder, esophageal and probably lung.

CHAPTER 7:

BIG WOMEN: BIG, BEAUTIFUL AND HEALTHY?

With apologies to Big Women, I really do not find overweight women sexy. I was certainly not considered sexy as a 228 pound, middle-aged Dad, with my belly hanging over my belt and my fat jowls framing a fat, Charlie Brown head. Everyone seems to agree, that fat guys are not sexy, so why is being a "big woman", "large woman" or "oversized woman" considered beautiful and sexy? I, and all of the men that I have asked, all agree, that the late Anna Nicole was very sexy looking as playmate of the year, when she weighed around a hundred pounds, but not so much when she was pushing two hundred pounds.

Mountains of credible research show that people are attracted to other healthy looking people. Men, world-wide, are attracted to women with a shape; women who have a small waist, hips and chest that are in proportion. Women prefer men who looked masculine, muscular, with flat abdomens, a "V" shape, large shoulders and small waist. In one study, the masculine appearance of the men preferred by the females, correlated exactly with the men who had "superior sperm", potentially the healthiest mates.

While driving early in the mornings in Coronado, California, Gayne and I would frequently encounter the Navy SEALS on their morning 5 mile run. These SEALS were in elite shape, running by in their skimpy little shorts, no shirts, wearing white socks and boots. Hoards of little "stud muffins", running in front of us, all buffed and sweaty. Gayne would say, "Stop the car, and don't talk, I just want to look." Sometimes she would even clean the windshield as they ran by. She would get a strange faraway look on her face, and sigh as they ran out of sight, and then she would lament, "I can remember when you used to look like that."

"What is the difference between a mistress and a wife?" "About 30 pounds". Gayne's comeback is, "What is the difference in a husband and a lover?" "About 40 pounds and 30 minutes". Both of these jokes have a disturbing ring of truth to them.

Recent studies of married couples, together longer than 15 years highlighted the emergence of the "DINS" (dual income no sex couples). Some 16% of long term married couples fail to have sex even once a month, and are very likely to be unhappy with their marriage and are more likely to get divorced. A reason for the declining frequency of sex in long-term marriages is not really clear. Perhaps familiarity really does breed contempt, or could it be the excessive weight of both partners? Is it possible that they might find their overweight partners less desirable?

Gayne and I were two married obese people sitting at home watching DVD's of Brad Pitt and Nicole Kidman. We would marvel at how good the movie stars looked, vicariously enjoying their sexuality, while fighting over that last few potato chips. I know, you can't hold yourself to that movie star standard, but we finally realized that we could look a lot sexier if we attained ideal body weight and toned our bodies. However, knowing that was not enough. But discovering that our obesity would lead diseases that would very likely prematurely kill us got our attention. Knowing that such diseases would cause incredible suffering and pain, and prevent us from seeing our future grandchildren grow up, was enough to get us started.

I am always mystified when I take care of an obese patient in the emergency room by their total lack of insight about the real disease threatening their lives. They are referred to as "land whales" by the emergency room staff, and they are frequently worried about the most insignificant problems, like a mild rash. "I just wanted to make sure it was not something serious, like cancer" They have a disease, "serious like cancer" but just don't know it.

The obese patient sits there, all 240 pounds of them, worried about a rash, when they really do have a disease as lethal as cancer, staring them in the face They complain about their debilitating low back pain, knee pain, fibromyalgia, migraine headaches, chronic fatigue syndrome, depression and chronic insomnia. They do not think any of these health problems have anything to do with their excessive weight.

Their overweight doctor has told them the perfunctory "lose weight and exercise", mantra and then started them on multiple medications that will only slow the tsunami of diseases and cause them to become narcotic and psychotropic drug addicts. The diseases will slowly overwhelm them, causing unimaginable suffering and disability and kill them early. I know that in the near future that I will be seeing them again, frequently, for life-threatening, true emergencies as they spiral down the drain.

If these obese patients are female, they are frequently advocates of the "Big and Beautiful" philosophy, and usually have a $500 hairdo, $60 nails, expensive makeup, shoes and lingerie. They must care how they look, but seem oblivious of the fact that attaining an ideal weight would make them look better than anything else they can do. It is sad to witness, because they have been told its ok to be "big", to accept your extra fat and to feel good about yourself. They always seem to continue to gain more weight, and then develop the domino effect of diseases and suffering and that will soon render them invalids. When that happens their only goal in life becomes trying to stay alive and trying to relieve their incessant pain and suffering.

It is useless to debate the question of whether obese women are beautiful and sexy; it's in the eye of the beholder. I have asked numerous women to name a fat guy that they thought was sexually attractive, "Please just name one fat, sexy man." No sincere answers so far, including their overweight husbands. The reason that the late Teddy Kennedy had to chase women around in his extra-large, ill-fitting boxer shorts is because they did not want to sleep with him.

There seems to be a double standard. The obese celebrity women who push the "Big and Beautiful" notion to the public say its "ok" to be obese. The number of adolescent females with excessive weight, especially in Blacks and Hispanics, is epidemic. These young females are already starting to develop metabolic syndrome, and the cascade of diseases leading to premature hypertension, cardiovascular disease, precious puberty, and cancers. Telling this young population that is ok to be obese, is irresponsible, and ignores the fact that it is dangerous and unhealthy to be obese.

Those "Big and Beautiful" women deserve a chance to extend their functional life span. Where are the "thousand woman" walks to raise consciousness and funds to fight obesity, or heart disease, the number one killer of women? Being overweight or obese is not healthy; women need to understand that it is much more than an acceptance of appearance or a vanity issue.

CHAPTER 8:

SMOKING: YOU CAN'T BE SERIOUS

NO SMOKING

Let's get this insanity out of the way. Before talking about the self-destructive idiocy of smoking, let me save you the trouble of giving me all of your excuses; "too much stress", "wrong time", "will gain weight", "will be testy", "plan to quit pretty soon", "have cut down", "plan to try some patches, bracelets, crystals, electronic cigarettes" or a new "anti-smoking diet" you heard about. And, oh yeah, you heard about someone "who smoked two packs a day and lived to be 103 years old".

Smoking is associated with early death, depending on the pack years (packs x years of smoking), with the average of 15 to 17 years lost by two pack a day habit. Long term smoking always leads to the development of predictable lung disease including; chronic bronchitis, emphysema, or chronic obstructive pulmonary disease or COPD (a kind of combination of both). Many types of cancers are associated with smoking, the most obvious being lung cancer (the number one cancer killer of women), gastric cancer, esophageal cancer, bladder cancer pharyngeal/laryngeal cancer, and many more yet to be linked.

If I wanted to really torture someone, to make their life a living hell, I would give them chronic obstructive lung disease. If you have known someone who died of chronic end-stage emphysema, you have seen the real suffering of end stage COPD patients. You have seen Hell on earth. They smother to death for a period of several years. Any small lung infection or flu can kill them. They are dependent on nebulizer machines and tethered to those little oxygen machines, 24 hours a day. They must use up to 8 or more very expensive medicines multiple times daily, just to keep breathing. They cannot walk across the room without getting short of breath, much less travel, or have any exertional physical activity, including sex.

If you want to know what COPD feels like, there are two ways that I demonstrate to my patients what it really feels like to have COPD.

In the first: take as deep a breath as you can and hold it in. Do Not Let It Out! Hold it for 45 seconds by the clock. Now, *without letting the breath out*, hold it in, breath "on top of "the held breath". That's the problem with COPD: air is trapped in damaged lung tissue, and it decreases the amount of air that can be taken in for oxygenation.

In the second: get a standard drinking straw the next time you are in the convenience store or burger stand. Put the straw in your mouth. Now, pinch your nose and breathe through the straw only. After less than a minute it becomes a full-time job just to breath. Makes you wonder how that Indian could stay hidden so long, under water in the creek breathing through that reed? That horrible feeling of not getting enough air is called dyspnea, and it is always a constant symptom of COPD.

Perhaps most importantly, smoking is a huge risk factor for atherosclerotic cardiovascular disease (ASCVD). If you have any risk factors like positive family history, abnormal lipids, hypertension, diabetes or pre-diabetes, and of course, obesity, then smoking is like putting gasoline on the fire. It will accelerate your ASCVD and will almost guarantee that you will have a cardiovascular event, such as a massive heart attack, congestive heart failure, stroke, or sudden death, much sooner and more frequently than your age and risk matched peers, who do not smoke.

Many of my female patients claim that they smoke very little, "only at parties" or "just one or two cigarettes a day". Bad news, recent studies of women who are "light smokers" confirm the fact that they are three times more likely to drop dead from a heart attack than those women who do not smoke. In over 50% of the cases, the first sign of cardiovascular disease in these women was sudden death. Heart attack is the number one killer of women in the United States. There is hope. Women who stop smoking decrease their risk for sudden death over time, and after twenty years of abstinence have the identical risk as women who have never smoked. Enough said, just stop.

Take the time to observe the hardened smokers at work. Hopefully, they have been confined to some outside smoking area, or in some type of smoke-proof structure that allows tactful observation of this miserable group of self-destructive outcasts. Wander by and take a look. What you will see are guilty looking people, coughing, with wrinkled, aging skin. Smoking decreases the blood supply to the face, thins the skin, and accelerates wrinkling. There is a sick, kind of sallow color to their skin. Smoking makes you sick, makes you look sick and makes you look older. Sorry, John Boehner and President Obama, but it is what it is.

There are medications that can aid a smoker who has decided to really quit. This is a good thing, because the addiction is very tenacious, and has been compared to that of heroin addiction. In addition to the nicotine products like the patches and gum, there are some antidepressant medications that have been associated with decreased nicotine craving in a significant number of smokers. The best known is buptopion, or Wellbutrin, an older antidepressant, that is a weak inhibitor of dopamine uptake in the brain. It should not be given to people with a known seizure disorder, or with certain other types of other medications. Ask your physician about using the drug to decrease your nicotine craving, when you are truly committed to quitting.

There is some good news for smokers who cannot quit. If you adapt THE BATTLE BUDDY DIET, life-style, you will statistically out live your fellow smokers who are sedentary. Unfortunately, there is no diet, or exercise program that can stop the development and progression of COPD. So maybe you will just live longer and be sicker longer. Why not stop right now.

CHAPTER 9:

FOOD, CALORIES, EXERCISE, RESISTANCE TRAINING

FOOD AND CALORIES: THE BASICS

Calories are a measure of metabolic energy. Metabolic energy is needed for all of the functions of our bodies. Think of calories as the fuel for all of the important, life-sustaining functions of the body. We measure how much energy a certain food, in a certain amount, will supply in calories (actually kilocalories). Some types of foods can supply more energy than others, and are higher in calories than others. Fat provides 9 K calories per gram, while carbohydrates and protein each provide 4 K calories per gram. Alcohol is about 7 K calories per gram, with absolutely no nutrient value.

Excess energy, is caused by taking in more calories than we burn each day, and results in the storage of this excess energy or excess calories as fat. As far as body weight goes, it does not matter where the calories come from; you could live on cheese cake and cheese burgers, and stay thin. You just couldn't eat very much of them. On such a diet you would still be at risk for cardiovascular disease, even with an ideal weight, because the wrong diet will increase intravascular inflammation. As discussed earlier, Intravascular and cellular inflammation may be more important than blood lipid levels in predicting risk for heart attack and stroke.

THE BODY IS THE PERFECT BANK: IT NEVER MISSES A DEPOSIT!

It took me 60 years, despite a medical education, to really accept the fact that if I ate only 6 or 7 of my kids' French fries, the 60 calories were always deposited into my body fat "bank account". Either I had to burn them, or cut down on other calories to avoid an excess. But, I never did, because those calories really didn't count. If I had such a small dietary indiscretion, it really didn't matter, because tomorrow I'm going to exercise more and eat less. Yeah, that's the ticket!

So the only way to gain weight is to consume more calories than you metabolize. Which leaves us with the painful, sobering conclusion that the only way to lose weight is to burn more calories that you consume.

Around 3,500 excessive calories deposited equals one pound of fat. If you exercised enough in one session to burn 3,500 calories, you would lose one pound of body weight. In order to burn that amount of calories by exercise, one would need to be an elite athlete, capable of many hours of intense exercise, like the Iron Man Triathlon.

A better way, to permanently loose the weight, is to cut down your calculated daily calorie requirements by 500 calories a day. Thus, to get rid of one pound, it would take 7 days, one week, 500 calories x 7days for a loss of 3500 calories, or one pound. The process can be accelerated by adding regular exercise and weight lifting. We experienced more like two pounds a week weight loss, while on THE BATTLE BUDDY DIET program.

There are multiple web sites that will help you calculate your total daily calorie requirements, but approximate requirements are: an inactive person needs around 13 calories per pound of body weight a day, while a moderately active person would require around 16 calories per pound, and a very active person would need around 18 calories per pound. On average most women require around 1,400 to 1,600 calories a day, while men (because of greater muscle mass) usually require 2,200 to 2,800 calories a day. Notice that the requirements are based on body weight, so as you lose weight, you need fewer calories.

Since people's daily food intake is most influenced by the weight/volume of the food, the trick with a healthier, whole food, diet is to eat large volumes of low calorie; water rich, nutritious foods that make you feel full. We know that women eat about 3 pounds of food a day, men around 4 to 5 pounds. If that food is calorie rich, unhealthy food, you will continue to gain weight because you will not feel full and eat more.

THE BATTLE BUDDY DIET is simple: heavy in whole grains, and vegetables, beans and greens, fish and healthy fats. This diet is for life, and for the rest of your life. It maintains healthy weight, extends life and prevents disease. It is low in fat and animal protein. This diet allows you to eat large volumes of great tasting foods, with great nutrition, while losing weight, improving your blood lipids, blood pressure, and lessening your chance of cancer. It is truly a diet for life, the only one that works to keep weight off, extend life and insure independence.

This means that just 100 calories a day extra, in excess of your daily requirements (a small bagel, donut, soft drink, or handful of candy) will result in a 10 pound weight gain in one year. If you have been a couple for 10 years, you both may be 100 pounds overweight.

EXERCISE

I was a fat guy in great shape, frustrated by my insidious weight gain, expanding waist, creeping blood pressure, pre-diabetes and disappointing blood lipids. I expected exercise to control my weight, but even doing more, 7days a week, just did not stop the waistline creep. Only when I counted my calories and decreased them to 500 calories below daily requirements did the sustained weight loss start. Combining vigorous exercise with THE BATTLE BUDDY DIET will greatly accelerate the weight loss process, make you feel better, increase your energy levels and tone your body.

It takes vigorous exercise, for a least one hour, seven days a week to burn a significant amount of calories, or to benefit physiologically. The older people you see walking the malls, at slow pace, for thirty minutes 5 days a week will benefit from the exercise but will not lose weight. At a very slow pace they only burn around 650 calories a week, which means that it would take a month to lose a little less than one pound. However, if these same people exercised vigorously, walking for one hour, seven days a week, they would burn 2450 calories a week, or almost three pounds a month.

It is obvious that if that same exercise schedule is combined with a 500 calorie a day deficit, the total loss for 4 weeks would be almost eight pounds, or a two pound weight loss per week. That is what we both experienced.

The other benefits of regular vigorous exercise are longevity and a lesser incidence of ASCVD, even in matched patients with other risk factors, like smoking. Exercise has been shown to decrease depression, increase energy levels, lower blood pressure, and even improve blood lipids. Other long term study have shown that regular exercise decreases dementia, stroke, premature death of all causes, cancers, and has been shown to delay osteoporosis, help improve arthritis, and to preserve muscle mass with aging.

Finally, regular exercise is a critical part of weight maintenance; it is really hard to keep the weight off without exercise. It seems that regular exercise helps correct our normal dietary indiscretions like the 100 calories of chips you ate, or that mocha coffee. It allows a margin when you exceed your daily calorie requirements.

RESISTANCE TRAINING

"Pumping iron" at all ages is now acceptable and encouraged. Resistance training has many benefits, not the least of which is burning more calories. It has been shown that weight training increases lean tissue mass, muscle, which burns an additional 30 to 40 calories per day per pound of muscle. After age 30, you will lose about 1/3 pound of muscle a year. In fact, it is disturbing to learn that beginning at around age 60, muscles that are not stressed may lose their neural connections, atrophy, and become useless.

Resistance training has been shown to preserve muscle mass in older people, upwards of 80 to 90 % can be saved and even strengthened. Intense resistance training has been shown to increase general body metabolism for as long as two days, and burns just as many calories as intense aerobic exercise, like running at 70% intensity. Old age disability is greatly decreased by weight training. I would like to be able to get up out of a chair on my own at age 80, but will not be able to unless I maintain my quadriceps muscles.

Regular resistance training is important when dieting since you want to preserve muscle and stimulate muscle growth by stressing your muscles and eating extra protein. As you lose weight, not only will fat be burned, but some muscle protein will be broken down and used as energy. So to preserve muscle mass, muscles must be stressed, trained and fed.

Resistance training makes you look better quickly, when combined with optimal body weight. Women who lift weights do not look like men; they have beautiful shaped arms, legs, butt, and back. Gayne wanted to get rid of her "old lady jelly upper arms". After only six weeks of working on her upper arms and triceps, people at work noticed the improvement and started borrowing her weights to work on their own arms. Today she has arms like Michelle Obama.

There are many ways to accomplish resistance or stress training such as: free weights, weight machines, or using your own body weight in exercises such as Yoga, Pilates or Core training. Another great way is by using elastic tubes or "stretch cords". You can even use isometric exercises stressing your muscles against each other. Many gyms now cater to older clients and help them safely learn to use free weights and weight machines. Studies have shown that people over 60 to 90 years old can actually gain muscle mass and increase their strength by greater than 30% with regular resistance training.

Balance and flexibility should be built into your exercise program. There are numerous sources for finding an exercise/weight lifting programs. The federal government has several web sites with instructions on how to begin and sustain resistance training and exercise, and of course, the men's fitness magazines are an excellent source of how to train.

Certified personal trainers are a good bet if chosen carefully, and you like their style. Calorie counts for a variety of exercises, from running to gardening are available on many of these health internet sites, as apps for your phone or in your local book store.

To succeed in adapting to <u>THE BATTLE BUDDY DIET</u> program, you must only do FIVE simple things:

1. Avoid the lethal foods

2. Eat the right diet in the right amount

3. Exercise/resistance training 1 hour, seven days a week

4. Sleep at least 8 hrs. a night.

CHAPTER 10:

BASICS OF WEIGHT LOSS

MUST TAKE IN LESS FOOD (CALORIES) THAN YOU BURN (METABOLIZE) EACH DAY.

REGULAR EXERCISE AIDS WEIGHT LOSS, AND MAKES IT POSSIBLE TO KEEP THE WEIGHT OFF.

TO LOSE ONE POUND, YOU MUST ELIMINATE 3,500 CALORIES, FROM YOUR BODY EITHER THROUGH EXERCISE OR DIET, OR BOTH.

THAT MEANS TO LOSE A POUND A WEEK, YOU MUST HAVE A DEFICIT OF 500 CALORIES A DAY.

ANY STARVATION, FASTING WEIGHT LOSS PROGRAM, OR SPECIAL PREPACKAGED DIETS, WILL NEVER SUSTAIN WEIGHT LOSS.

LIFE-LONG SUSTAINED WEIGHT CONTROL REQUIRES A PERMANET CHANGE IN LIFE-STYLE, AND.DIET.

AVOIDING "BAD"FATS, SIMPLE CARBOHYDRATES, PROCESSED FOODS SUGARS AND LIMITING EXCESSIVE INTAKE IS THE KEY TO HEALTHY EATING AND SUSTAINED WEIGHT LOSS.

SUCCESS TOTALLY DEPENDS ON SELF-DISCIPLINE, COMMITMENT AND ON DEVELOPING NEW HEALTHY HABITS.

CHAPTER 11:

12 LETHAL FOODS

No Flour or any bread products made from processed grain, i.e. flour, are truly lethal. If the ingredients include the word "flour", do not buy it. The only allowable breads are the whole grain types, usually dark and heavy. It must state "whole grain". Watch out for misleading terms like, "cracked wheat", "multi-grain" and "whole wheat". No pasta, pizza or pie crust, oriental noodles, lasagna, tortillas, or sandwich wraps, unless they are truly whole grain. Whole grain breads, pastas, and crackers are available and will get better as demand increases.

No "Bad Fats" such as Beef, Pork or any type of mammal meat (except game meat). If it has fur, eyes, and a mother do not eat it. Do not eat it if it has feathers and comes from an egg. No poultry. No Trans-Fatty Acids. Heated, processed fat produces a type of alien fat, not found in nature called "Trans-fatty acids" or "Trans- fats". Trans-fats are man-made poison, not found in nature. They are added to food products, to make them solid, with a longer shelf-life, and a higher boiling point. Trans-fats have become a staple ingredient of processed cakes, donuts, cookies, chips, margarine and almost all processed snack foods, in the US and world-wide. Recent legislation requires manufactures to list Trans-fat content on nutrition labels. Another term used for Trans-fatty acids is "hydrogenated fats". If you see the words: Trans-fats, Trans-fatty acids, or "hydrogenated" anything, do not buy it or eat it. The bottom line: eat no processed foods!

No Fast Food, (Almost) Never! If you are forced into a fast food joint, look for a low/no fat salad with low fat, vegetable oil dressing, or balsamic vinegar. Many of these franchises are finally waking up and experimenting with "healthy salads", yogurt and berries, etc. Watch out for creamy dressing, and lethal animal fats, like ham, bacon, or beef mixed in salads and no croutons. Ask to see the nutritional information on the salad, and for an alternate dressing. A build-your-own sub sandwich, using whole grain bread, or "vegie burger", salmon burger, or portabella mushroom and low calorie dressing is a reasonable alternative. Healthy, easily available, fast whole foods will be a reality in the near future as the demand increases.

No Dairy Fat. No Dairy products. Sorry about the ice cream! Dairy fats are lethal fats. They are also highly caloric. Included in "bad" dairy foods are: cottage cheese, whipped cream, sour cream, ice cream, regular yogurt, creamy cheeses and milk. All of these foods are available in "no fat" versions, but they still have high calories and are poor sources of protein and are loaded with simple sugars. Beware of the "nondairy" coffee creamers, they are chemical poisons. The only dairy product that is acceptable is fat free, sugar free natural yogurt. You can sweeten it with Splenda.

No Fried Foods of any type and that especially includes: the so-called "vegetable", French fries. Deep-fried anything, tempura, pan fried foods, donuts, funnel cake, hash browns, and fried seafood are absolutely lethal. It is permissible to use very small amounts of vegetable based cooking oils, like canola or olive oil, to sear seafood, or to stir-fry fresh vegetables.

No Baked Goods Watch out for the "low fat muffin", or the "fat free cookies", they frequently have a heavy carbohydrate load, flour, sugar, and are highly caloric. Crackers, cookies, pretzels, cupcakes, and baked chips are lethal. Sorry about the old standby, the bagel, and forget about the cinnamon buns. Baked "whole grain" products are available, but watch the carbohydrates and sugars. "Healthy" baked anything is really an oxymoron. The exception is genuine whole grain bread or cookies.

No Sugared Soft Drinks or fruit Juices. They are high in sugar (20 grams!) or fructose (a simple, deadly sugar), sodium and have lots of empty calories. Chemically sweetened, non-carbonated drinks are permissible in moderation, like Crystal Lite. Avoid bottled juices, sodas of any kind, "energy" or "power" drinks, including "mixed" fruit juices. Never drink any fruit juices, even unsweetened, including orange juice; they are highly caloric, even unsweetened, and lack the fiber provided by eating the fruit itself. Eat fruit, don't drink it. Carbonated drinks, like sugar-free sodas are lethal since because of their phosphorus content, they leech calcium out of bones and accelerate osteoporosis.

No Alcohol or Strictly Limit Intake to two ounces a day or less, and make it red wine. As we all know, two glasses of red wine a day has been shown to decrease fatal heart attack risk. It is the dark grape in red wine that provides clotting protection, not the alcohol. More than two ounces of red wine a day does not offer any additional benefit. Better to limit it to two drinks a week or none at all. Remember, an ounce of alcohol contains significant calories, and will stimulate appetite and bad dietary decisions. Alcohol is metabolized preferentially, and causes the metabolism of other foods, eaten at the same time, to go into fat storage. We like to forget that alcohol is a poison.

No Animal Fat, Saturated Cooking Oils especially lard and butter, high in saturated fats. Avoid coconut oil, peanut oil, and corn oil. Use canola oil or olive oil in very small amounts for cooking. Forget saving the bacon fat, or cooking with fatback. Especially lethal are the white sauces made with butter.

No milk, even fat free milk, since it contains a high carbohydrate and sugar load (12 grams), in an 8 oz. glass, and is highly caloric (90 calories). Try flavored soy milk, or almond milk, it tastes better and is healthier, and can be found in a low fat, low carb variety and is frequently fortified with extra calcium. Soy consumption has been linked to longevity, decreased risk of heart disease and optimal weight maintenance.

No White rice or White Potatoes use brown rice and yams instead. White rice and white potatoes are high calorie sources of simple carbohydrates. They have very little nutritional value, and are rapidly absorbed, causing insulin surges, which stimulate hunger, and shift metabolism towards storage of calories as fat.

No Sweets, Candy or Pastry Desserts including: milk chocolate (mixed with sugar and milk), candy, crepes, pies, cheese cake, fruit tarts, pastries, fruit cobbler, ice cream and the ubiquitous donut holes. Any food made with sugar is not needed by your body, and should be avoided. Sugar is super lethal, addictive and directly linked to the development of diabetes and obesity. No sugar, ever! Dark chocolate, or semi-sweet, is acceptable and may even be beneficial in altering mood, especially in women and provides lycopenes and antioxidants to combat aging.

CHAPTER 12:

DIET FOR LIFE

WHAT YOU SHOULD EAT FOR THE REST OF YOUR LIFE

After thousands of years of man subsisting on grains, plants, legumes, roots, berries, fruits, fish, and rarely, game meat, modern man has evolved a diet completely foreign to our alimentary tracts, in just the last five generations. Modern man has adapted the "Western Diet"; one high in animal fats, dairy fats, sweets, simple carbohydrates, and processed foods.

Specific "lethal" ingredients found in the Western Diet include: simple sugars (glucose, fructose), fruit juices, animal saturated (bad) fats, oils, Trans-fats (synthetic, very bad fats), and dairy products, especially cow's milk. All of these delicious, but lethal foods are supplied to our diets by ubiquitous, highly processed foods, candy and sweets, animal fats (beef and pork), and high fat, high sugar dairy products.

Yes, many lethal foods that we have learned to love and to eat in abundance, are everywhere. Access to such a diet does not involve hunting and gathering, it merely requires opening the pantry, glove compartment, or refrigerator, calling pizza delivery or pulling into a fast food outlet. The "Western Diet" is decimating the health of our society, at all ages, and most tragically, is leading to a pandemic of obesity linked diseases in children.

All children and adults, who continue to eat this diet, will gain weight, and once above a BMI of 25 (overweight) to 30 (obesity), or greater, will have a massively increased risk for adult obesity linked diseases and premature death. There are now some 38 diseases linked to Western diet induced obesity. The most common are: diabetes, hypertension, lipid disorders, cancers, stroke, asthma, cardiovascular disease (ASCVD), and dementia. They all cause functional disability, resulting in total dependency on chronic medical care just to sustain life, and ultimately to a painful, disease-riddled early death.

Your Grandmother was right! You should eat more whole, unprocessed, foods like vegetables, grains, fruits and fish. In long-term study after study, involving thousands of patients, followed for 30 years or more, with all other risk factors matched: those people who ate a "prudent" diet;

one with more vegetables, grains, fruit and fish, and fewer animal fats, dairy products and processed foods, lived significantly longer (around 10 to 12 years average) than those who did not. Not only do these people live significantly longer, they live a more self-sufficient, functional, independent, active, and "happier" life.

THE BATTLE BUDDY DIET is a prudent diet, unique because it forbids all lethal foods, and advocates a mix of only healthy whole foods and fish. A prudent diet, and optimal body weight, has absolutely been shown to eliminate disability in aging adults, by preventing, or even reversing the devastating, metabolic and cardiovascular co-morbid diseases directly related to obesity and the Western Diet. Healthy, active, older people who keep their weight in the normal range and eat a prudent diet are functional, independent, mentally sharp, and happier than their sick cohorts.

There is no question that adults using a whole food, prudent diet are more likely to have ideal body weight, to be more active, mobile, alert, sexually active and less depressed. That is because they are not ill or suffering, not "umbilicated" to chronic medical care, dependent on multiple medications, machines, and other people, just to stay alive.

Prudent diet and ideal body weight separate the healthy active aging adults from the chronically ill, disabled, adults. Ideal body weight and prudent diet insure greater functional longevity by dramatically decreasing or even reversing the incidence of diabetes, hypertension, high bad lipids, atherosclerotic cardiovascular disease, ASCVD (coronary artery disease, stroke, and atherosclerotic vascular disease), crippling arthritis, chronic back disc problems, asthma, and growing list of cancers, most dramatically, colon cancer, prostate cancer, breast and lung cancer.

The foundation of this diet is the regular intake of whole foods: grains, vegetables, fruits, nuts, and fish. Man-made food products, processed foods, simple sugars, animal and dairy foods are lethal and are to be absolutely avoided.

A prudent diet has the advantage of making you feel full, since you can eat great amounts of "beans and greens", vegetables, and grains with many fewer calories, and more nutritional value than the calorie dense foods of the Western Diet. Multiple studies have shown that men and women eat a constant daily amount of food based on volume and weight, with the average man eating 4 to 5 lbs. a day and a women consistently eat around 3 lbs.

"Volumetric", water-rich foods like vegetables, beans, healthy soups, fruits, and grains, can supply satisfying volume, a feeling of being "full", and complete nutrition.

A whole food prudent diet's major benefit is that it supplies required daily vitamins and minerals and a multitude of healthy, powerful substances found in vegetables and grains called phytonutrients; such as the carotenoids, flavonoids, lycopenes and other "anti-aging" and anticancer, antioxidants. These substances have been shown to help prevent diabetes, cancers, ASCVD, macular degeneration of the eye, and have been shown to slow the cellular aging process.

Most recently, there are exciting studies that show that a low fat, low carbohydrate diet, high in soy protein, vegetables, fruits and grains, is equal to a "statin" cholesterol lowering drug in reducing bad cholesterol and increasing good cholesterol in a small group of men. Most internists and cardiologists tend to push medications, because diet and exercise "always fail", and there is almost no reimbursement in recommending diet and lifestyle changes. Patients want a magic pill that "cures" their disease and allows them to continue their self-destructive lifestyle. I think recommending diet and exercise do not work because neither the physician nor the patient know how important it is, to really adapt a permanent diet and lifestyle change, Instead, we are looking for a quick fix, a "magic pill" or unsustainable crash diet to cure us.

Furthermore, there is now unprecedented, objective research showing that endogenous self-repair of atherosclerotic arteries is possible with strict adherence to this whole food, prudent diet. Published reports of "hopeless", even "inoperable" cases of coronary artery disease patients, placed on this strict whole foods diet, have shown, by objective coronary angiograms, to reverse their blockages, by self-repairing the endothelium or lining of their coronary arteries. One of the plausible theoretical explanations is that many of the Omega-3 foods (nuts, fish) increase intravascular nitric oxide. Nitric oxide is important in maintaining blood flow through arteries, makes platelets less "sticky" (prevents blood clots), and seems to directly repair the inflammatory plaques of ASCVD.

Vegetables and whole grain foods are rich sources of protein, minerals and vitamins, and supply the greatest amount of nutrition with the fewest calories. They supply complete nutrition, complex carbohydrates, and the all-important, fiber.

Fiber is that part of the food that is not totally absorbed by the bowels. Fiber is found in vegetables, grains and fruits and is critical to proper bowel function. Intake of significant dietary fiber has been shown to decrease the incidence of colon, prostate, and breast cancer. In multiple studies, high fiber intake is associated with optimal body weight (BMI), less diabetes, hypertension and abnormal lipids.

The complex carbohydrates are absorbed from the gut slowly and in a complex form that requires more metabolism to break them down into simple sugars. A simple or refined carbohydrate, like the flour found in your morning bagel, will be broken down quickly, causing a sugar surge in the blood that stimulates insulin release. Refined or simple carbohydrates, like glucose, are said to have a high "glycemic index", and will cause insulin surges, and insulin insensitivity, the precursor of acquired (type II) diabetes.

This insulin surge, even when the level returns to normal, stimulates hunger. That is why after eating your breakfast bagel, or muffin, you get famished at 10:30 am every day, wondering why it's not lunch time yet. This insulin response is blunted, by eating complex carbohydrates, like grains and vegetables, and subsequently decreases the chance of developing acquired diabetes (Type II).

The foundations of <u>THE BATTLE BUDDY DIET</u> are whole foods, vegetables and whole grain foods. These are the foods that require a reacquisition of your primitive tastes. You must learn to prefer them over the lethal foods. The benefits are immense!

REMEMBER, IF IT IS PROCESSED FOOD, OR MAN-MADE, DO NOT EAT IT! IF IT HAS FUR, FEATHERS OR IS WHITE, DO NOT EAT IT! IF IT IS FRIED, OR HAS SIMPLE SUGAR IN IT, DO NOT EAT IT.

<u>THE BATTLE BUDDY DIET</u>

<u>THE BATTLE BUDDY DIET</u> consists of only 4 large food groups: (1) Grains and Cereals, (2) Vegetables, (3) Fruits, (4) Protein, nuts and healthy fats. Vitamins and supplemental nutrients are not usually needed and not recommended, this diet supplies all that is needed for healthy adults and children.

GRAINS AND CEREALS: 6 (or more), SERVINGS/DAY

It is our belief, based on credible scientific support, that eating 6 or more servings of whole grains a day is a key ingredient of successful, sustained weight loss, functional, quality, longevity and a healthier body at any age. Let's think, what did primitive man eat, that kept him alive, free of cancer and able to evolve? He ate mostly grains, plant derived foods, seeds, berries, legumes, and roots.

The primitive men that have been recovered from ice or bogs, have two things in common: first, what was recovered from their stomachs; grains, beans, and berries, some with fish, or jerky made from game; second, all of these mummies were elite physiologic beings at the time of death. They were in great shape! They had no signs of any of the obesity related diseases or cancers that are ubiquitous in our society. They had no need for an aerobics or Pilates class, or a nature walk, they were active just trying to stay alive. As you already know, exercise is the other mandatory, key ingredient of a functional longevity.

The term "whole grain" means just that; the entire seed, husk and all, is used in the product. The husk, or outer covering of the grain, is the source of all of the healthy nutrients and a great source of fiber.

On the nutrition labels of a grain product, like bread, the use of the term, "whole grain" should mean that the grain, like wheat, is in the product unchanged. Beware of the term, "whole grain flour", that is an oxymoron. "Flour" anywhere in the ingredients means the food is not the unaltered whole grain. "Whole Grain" should be the first ingredient listed, so look specifically for the term "whole grain", but be careful of other ingredients, like added sugars and processed carbohydrates. To legally use the term, "whole grain", a product must contain at least 51% or more of whole grain by weight.

Whole grain healthy breads are usually dark and heavy; the kind that if you dropped a loaf on your foot, you might need an x-ray. But beware; bread can be made dark and heavy with dark sugars, and food coloring. The use of words like "multigrain", "stone ground", "cracked wheat", "seven grain" or "bran" are used to increase the "health appeal" of the bread, but they are not truly whole grain. If it does not say "whole grain", it is flour rich, processed bread and very unhealthy, in fact, processed bread, a simple carbohydrate, is on the lethal list.

Healthy types of whole grain foods include: oatmeal, whole grain bran, low fat/ low sugar whole grain cereals, brown rice, wild rice, quinoa, whole grain crackers, low fat popcorn, whole wheat products, whole rye, whole grain pastas, and wheat germ. Examples of servings of these foods, include: 1 slice of whole grain bread, one cup of cereal, ½ cup of brown rice, 5 whole grain crackers, 3 cups of popped popcorn, and 1 cup of oatmeal.

VEGETABLES 4 (or more) SERVINGS A DAY

The great thing about vegetables, besides them being so healthy, is that they are almost "free" in a prudent diet. Because they are so low in calories, you can have multiple servings, without exceeding your daily calorie allowance. They have the greatest volume, most fiber, and the highest water content, all of which make you feel full.

The darker the vegetable, the more nutrition it supplies. For example, regular iceberg lettuce is light in color and has almost no nutrient value. It is mostly only water. A delicious alternative is fresh spinach, or kale, both of which are absolutely loaded with minerals, vitamins and other valuable nutrients.

Almost all beans and peas (legumes) are excellent sources of fiber, complex carbohydrates, good fats, and a great source of plant protein. Be sure to get the kind that are not sweetened, or have added fat, like "pork and beans" or "re-fried beans". Beans have more calories than some other types of vegetables, but have the added benefit of supplying plant protein and essential fats. Legumes can be made into soups, another great way to increase the volume of healthy food and to feel full.

Vegetables should be a mainstay for healthy snacking. A handful of baby carrots (eat them one at a time), is only 38 calories, an excellent source of vitamin A, and can make you feel full. Any fresh vegetable, like broccoli, can be dipped in a no fat/low calorie dip, or olive oil based vinegar dressing, for a great, satisfying, mid-day or evening snack. Mushrooms are great sautéed, without oil, just use water to continue searing. This works with any vegetable and is great with a little salt and added spice.

A list of the best vegetables include: dark green leafy vegetables (spinach, kale, mustard greens, collards, romaine lettuce, and cabbage), broccoli, red cabbage, yams, orange or yellow squash, and lentils. Deep green, yellow and orange vegetables are always the most beneficial.

Carbohydrates are required for optimal metabolism and immediate energy needs. The carbohydrates that we crave, like processed bread, processed snacks, cakes, cookies, doughnuts, jams, jellies, soft drinks, white potato, white rice, refined breakfast cereal and even milk are all on the "lethal list". Vegetables are the best dietary source of starch and complex carbohydrates. We can get all of our necessary carbohydrates from grains and vegetables, which are far healthier, provide extra beneficial ingredients, blunt the insulin surge, and make us feel full.

Tomatoes deserve special mention. Tomatoes are really a fruit, but they seem more at home in the company of vegetables. Tomatoes of all types provide all of the good things, like fiber, vitamins and minerals, but in addition, provide powerful substances called lycopenes, that are super potent antioxidants, that slow cellular aging. Long term studies show a highly significant decrease in prostate cancer in men who eat tomatoes on a regular basis. Tomatoes in any form, from juice to tomato sauces, puree, or salsa are beneficial. Remember, the juice alone does not supply the fiber.

FRUITS 2 (or more) SERVINGS A DAY

Fruits should include all types, citrus, berries, apples, bananas and all the others. They are loaded with essential vitamins including A, C, and folic acid. Fruits are an important source of potassium (K+), an electrolyte critical in the normal functioning of muscles, including the heart muscle, both in pumping and in conduction or rhythm function. High K fruits include: apricots, prunes, oranges and, of course, bananas.

Fruits supply fiber, but only if eaten whole. Fruit juices should absolutely be avoided; they are on the "lethal list", because they are high in sugar content, calories, mostly water and supply fewer nutrients than the whole fruit. Stay with the fruits that are darker in color or orange and eat the fruit, never just drink the juice. Juicer machines short circuit the advantages of fiber, and limit feeling of fullness. Eat the fruit!

Some fruits have so much sugar or glucose in them (high glycemic index), and very little nutritional value that they should be avoided, in excess, such as: watermelon, grapes, dried apricots, raisins, and papaya. Watch out for the "low fat" trail mixes; they frequently have high calorie dried fruits, high calorie nuts, chocolate, sugar and sometimes, processed products. Always check the nutrition label prior to buying any "healthy" snack food.

The best kept secret in fruits is the berry. Your diet should have berries on a daily basis. You should include all types; blueberries, blackberries, raspberries, and of course, the old stand-by favorite, strawberries. They are loaded with healthy nutrients, potent antioxidants, complex carbohydrates and they provide fiber and vitamins.

Berries are relatively low in calories, and just as nutritious frozen or fresh. They make a great topping for a whole grain cereal mixed with fat-free yogurt, almond or soy milk. They are a quick healthy snack, or desert. They provide long term benefits, because they contain very potent antioxidants, shown to delay aging at the cellular level. I recommend at least two servings a day. Fresh berries are seasonal and can be expensive. The frozen ones are cheaper and just as nutritious. I like to eat them frozen on whole grain cereal, or with a little fat-free yogurt and a whole grain cereal.

PROTEIN/FAT (2 SERVING OR MORE, A DAY)

Protein is the only source of the critical building blocks of our bodies, the amino acids. There are twenty amino acids, eleven can be made by our bodies by breaking down our own protein, but the other nine are called "essential" and must be ingested. The essential amino acids are found in "complete" protein foods, such as, beans and fish.

Proteins are made up of linked amino acids, folded up in very specific sequences to perform multiple functions. Our body proteins are the basis of: enzymes, antibodies, hormones, muscle, genetic codes and DNA/RNA production, messengers to cells and immune system, and our hair and nails.

Mammalian animal meat, dead mammals, as a source of protein, has the grave disadvantage of being laden with very bad fats (highly saturated) and is highly caloric. Regular ingestion of animal fat (Western Diet) has been proven to be associated with obesity, ASCVD, cancers, abnormal blood lipids, stroke, and even lung disease. Animal meat is a rather poor source of quality protein, with some 40% of the amino acids consisting of glutamic acid, a non-essential amino acid. Animal fat is high on the "lethal foods" list, and should never be your source of protein.

Say goodbye to poultry. Yes, I too, thought that eating chicken breasts baked, without the skin, was acceptable and that turkey breast has always been allowed on most "healthy diets". After all, we need to eat it to get the protein, don't we? Sorry, but the poultry we get in the U.S. is grain fed and has the same drawbacks as mammalian meat; it is an incomplete protein source and loaded with harmful fats. We eat one million chickens an hour in the U.S. and they are loaded with Omega-6 and Omega-8 fats, which are harmful in excess. You can eat skinless duck, pheasant, or truly free-range chicken because the fat content shifts back towards Omega-3, the healthy fat.

Cooking oils should only be plant based, unsaturated vegetable oils (coconut and palm oil are lethal). The best are olive oil and canola oil. Avoid any hydrogenated cooking oils, animal based oils like lard, coconut oil, and butter since they are highly caloric and full of lethal saturated fats.

The best sources of protein are fish and plants. They are characterized by high quality protein and healthy, essential unsaturated fats ("Omega fats") necessary for critical cellular functions in the heart and brain. Regular consumption of certain types of fish (wild salmon) has been shown to be associated with significant increased longevity, decreased ASCVD and stroke, and a decreased incidence of prostate cancer in studies of over 50,000 adults, spanning 50 years or more.

Wild salmon is the fish of choice. It only has to be consumed two times a week to afford protection against ASCVD. Additional amounts of fish have not been shown to increase protection against ASCVD and early death. The Omega-3 fats in fish are incorporated, unchanged into our brain cells. They also decrease the incidence of blood clot associated with stroke and myocardial infarction (heart attack).

Other types of great fish sources are: most salt-water white fish, sardines, halibut, tuna, trout, shark and sword fish. Of course, no fish should ever be fried, and remember, a single serving is about the size of a standard index card. Fish and other sea foods can be caloric and should be eaten in moderation. Many contain high cholesterol levels, and there is some concern that the levels of Mercury in fish could endanger those who consume large amounts. This is not a real concern, except in pregnant women who should probably limit their fish intake.

If you must have meat other than fish, then it must be limited to game meat, or free-range bison. Again, never fried, and watch out for barbecue and marinate sauces (sugar/carbs).

Keep an open mind, and explore the world of Soy Tofu, a plant complete protein source, associated with increased longevity and improvement in blood lipids and decreased vascular inflammation. There are some great tasting tofu products that simulate burgers, spare ribs, and even ice cream. As always, read the ingredients, to make sure there are no added saturated fats or simple sugars. As the demand grows, I expect to see more competition for such products, and better tasting new soy based foods.

Free-range (not grain fed chickens) eggs are a great source of protein, but you do not need to eat the cholesterol laden, calorie rich, yolk. Have an egg-white omelet with vegetables. Most experts suggest limiting egg consumption to twice a week, if you are eating the yolk. Regular eggs, from grain fed chickens, are totally different, and are lethal.

Nuts, though high in calories, are an excellent source of the good fats (Omega-3) and have been shown to decrease the incidence of diabetes and ASCVD in multiple longevity studies. They tend to satiate hunger and make an excellent healthy snack, but only in moderation. A serving, (2 oz.), is only about 10-12 nuts, so you cannot grab handfuls. Cashews, almonds, walnuts and pecans are the best, and should be followed by 8 oz. of liquid to augment the full feeling.

High protein diets, with low carbohydrates, have been shown to accelerate weight loss and to preserve muscle mass. In <u>**THE BATTLE BUDDY DIET**</u> program, we recommend much more protein in the diet than most of the experts. The argument against a high protein diet has been that excessive protein could cause kidney failure. This is a myth. Normal people on an otherwise balanced diet, with adequate hydration, and no systemic diseases, do not develop kidney disease on a high protein diet.

Protein has fewer calories than fat, and has been found to be "thermo genic", meaning that it takes more energy for the body to process protein than simple carbohydrates. In this instance, not all calories are equal. Protein intake is associated with a more even blood sugar release, preventing the insulin surges that can lead to diabetes, and make us feel hungry.

Since this plan incorporates exercise and resistance training for life, it is essential to continue a relatively high protein intake. The rebuilding and repair of muscle requires protein. Building increased muscle mass increases our metabolic rate up to 15 fold, with each additional pound of muscle burning about 30 extra calories a day. Weight training requires protein to rebuild and grow muscle, especially while limiting calories.

WHY NOT DAIRY PRODUCTS?

"Have Milk?" I hope not. I say never! Cow's milk is truly lethal. There are even some nutritional experts who call milk a "carcinogen", and indeed, Casein, the major component of milk, has been shown to accelerate tumor growth in some animal cancer studies. What about "non-fat" milk? Read the ingredients, an 8 oz. glass has nearly the same simple sugar content and calories as a sugared soft drink! You should never drink cow's milk again, ever! And you should never feed it to your children!

As Arnold so eloquently stated in the movie "Pumping Iron", "Milk is for babies." But not really, babies should drink only breast milk or formula, cow's milk makes them fat and is unhealthy. Go to the refrigerator and get out the fat-free milk and read the nutrition label. You will be shocked to find that an 8oz. drinking glass has 90 calories, over 12 grams of simple sugar, and around 12 grams of carbohydrate, and only 30% of the daily calcium requirement. The most common reason for drinking milk that I hear is that it is needed for calcium. There are many other foods richer in calcium, and calcium is a frequent supplement added to cereals and soy and almond milk, which have fewer calories and more nutrition than cow's milk.

Calcium is needed by the body to aid muscle contraction, especially that of heart muscle, and is linked to the conduction system of the heart. It is essential for normal blood clotting, bone growth and repair, and has been shown in multiple studies that calcium intake accelerates weight loss. Cow's milk is a poor source of Calcium You can get all you need from plants, supplements and from soy or almond milk, especially if fortified with Calcium.

The fatty dairy products that we crave, like ice cream (my old favorite), cheese, sour cream, cream cheese, and mayonnaise, are all on the "lethal list". There are non-dairy substitutes for all of these products, some better than others. Nonfat yogurt, with no added sugar, is probably safe, and the only dairy food allowed on this diet. It is a great substitute for ice cream and can be sweetened with a safe sugar substitute, like Splenda.

Let's consider soy products and tofu. Before you say, no way, not "soy" stuff, because it's a kind of strange food those eccentric, holistic, vegan people eat. Real men eat beef! Besides, it's kind of slimy (think tofu), and it is not something most of us would choose to eat. That was in the old days. Now soy is available in good tasting foods, and as an added supplement. Soy in any form seems to be a powerhouse of nutritional plant protein, found to be associated with significantly reduced rates of ASCVD. Soy is the only plant protein containing all of the essential amino acids (those amino acids not made by the body).

One of our favorite drinks is soy milk. It is high protein juice squeezed from the intact soy bean. It can be flavored and fortified with minerals and calcium, and is available in a reduced fat form. It is very low in fat, carbohydrates, and sugar. It provides more high quality, essential protein, than cow's milk, and tastes great, cold, on a whole grain cereal, or as a "soy latte" at the coffee shop. Try it at least three times before you decide you cannot switch, it tastes richer than milk, and we love it.

Cheeses are suspect, but "ok", in moderation, but only the non-fat or low fat varieties. Low-fat is acceptable here, because non-fat cheese is sometimes just not eatable. Cheese is another good source of dietary calcium. Creamy cheeses like, Brie are not acceptable, and are considered "lethal". The healthiest cheeses are the "natural" cheeses, like: Swiss, Mozzarella, Cheddar, and Parmesan. Measure a serving, in a measuring cup, to get a feel for the amount of a serving. Not too much, it can be high in calories.

The "French Paradox", is the fact that in several studies, age-matched, risk-matched French people, who eat fat rich foods, suffered less ASCVD than their risk-matched American counterparts. Initially, this advantage was ascribed to the consumption of red wine, and indeed, that benefit continues to be borne out by the literature. However, there is now mounting evidence, that the consumption of cheese at the end of the meal, may physically bind some fatty foods keeping them from being fully absorbed.

THE BOTTOM LINE

Stick to **THE BATTLE BUDDY DIET** for life. Be rigorous about staying faithful to eating only the right foods and you will be rewarded by having less disease and a happier functional life. Some diets allow "cheating" so that you don't get "cravings". Switch your cravings to healthy foods, and don't cheat yourself and your body.

CHAPTER 13:

BAD DIETARY FATS (LETHAL)

SATURATED FATS

ANIMAL SOURCES

BEEF, PORK

TALLOW

LARD

VEGETABLE SOURCES

DAIRY FATS

PALM OIL

COCONUT OR COCONUT OIL

COCA BUTTER

<u>TRANS-FATS</u>

MARGARINE AND OTHER BUTTER SUBSITUTES

FRIED FOODS

PROCESSED BAKED GOODS

PROCESSED SNACK FOODS

<u>CHOLESTEROL</u> (NOT AS BAD IN SEAFOOD; OTHER POSITIVES)

DAIRY PRODUCTS WITH FAT

SHELL FISH, CRUSTATIONS

POULTRY SKIN AND DARK MEAT, EGG YOLKS

CHAPTER 14:

GOOD DIETARY FATS

MONOUNSTURATED FATS (OMEGA-9) GOOD

OILS

OLIVE OIL

CANOLA OIL

POLYUNSATURATED FATS (OMEGA-6, OMEGA-3) BETTER

OILS

CANOLA OIL

COTTON SEAD OIL

CORN OIL

SOYBEAN OIL

SUNFLOWER OIL

SAFFLOWER OIL

FISH

SALMON

SARDINES (IN WATER)

TUNA

SWORD FISH

OTHER WHITE FISH

VEGETABLES

NUTS   (WALNUTS,   MACADAMIAN,   CASHEW, OTHERS)

FLAXSEED AND OIL

RAPESEED AND OIL

SOY BEANS AND OIL

WHEAT GERM

CHAPTER 15:

GOALS FOR <u>THE BATTLE BUDDY DIET</u> PROGRAM

To achieve a BMI of 25 or less, or your best weight maintained for at least a year after the age of 20y.

Change your tastes to adopt a whole food, prudent, healthy diet for life.

Regain high energy and enthusiasm for life by embracing your healthy life style and the new you.

Prioritize and commit to life-long exercise for at least one hour daily, every day.

Commit to resistance training at least thirty minutes three days a week, for life.

Have optimal sleep each night, at least 8 hours as an adult

CHAPTER 16:

HOW TO START

COMMIT: "ALL IN"

Accept that you have too much body fat and that you eat the wrong foods, that this is unhealthy, and that it will shorten your life, make you suffer and make you sick. If you are a couple, you should both acknowledge your own individual problem with weight. Take responsibility for your body, but pledge to support each other, as true Battle Buddies. Rigorously adapt <u>THE BATTLE BUDDY DIET</u> program. Pledge to yourself and each other to give the program just 4 weeks.

MEDICAL EVALUATION

Get a baseline physician evaluation to include: your BMI, waist measurement, and a complete medical evaluation from your physician. That would include: appropriate blood tests (lipid profile,hs C-reactive protein in addition to usual blood work appropriate for age, sex) evaluation for exercise (stress cardiac evaluation) and resistance training (weights), and any other specialty procedures necessary, such as: colonoscopy, mammogram, or Pap smear.

BASELINE RECORDS

Record where you are with revealing dated pictures, full body, front, back and profile in a revealing bathing suit (no sucking it in). Record and save all of your blood tests results, lipid and C reactive protein levels, blood pressure and resting pulse. You should measure and record the circumference of your waist, thighs, hips, chest, and arms.

JETTISON THE JUNK

Clean all of the lethal foods out of your house, workplace and car. If it is left available, you will find it and eat it.

STOCK UP ON HEALTHY FOODS

Go shopping together, with your Battle Buddy and the kids for food and load up only on healthy recommended foods, and keep all lethal foods out of the basket.

SCHEDULE EXERCISE AND MAKE IT A PRIORITY

Schedule and prioritize your exercise. One hour of vigorous exertion, seven days a week. Remember, you can break it up into 15 min efforts throughout the day, or do it all at once. Calculate your calories expended, and log the data.

PUMP THE IRON

Prioritize resistance training, weights, or some other form and do at least 30 minutes, three days a week. Skip at least one day between weight training sessions. The 30 minutes counts towards your one hour of exercise a day.

MANAGE YOUR MEDICATIONS

If you are taking medicines for any chronic illness, check with your physician. As you drop your weight and exercise, you can usually be weaned off of medicines for hypertension, hyperlipidemia, and even diabetes.

WEIGH IN AND RECORD ONCE A WEEK

Weigh yourself once a week, on the same scale. You can calculate or measure your body fat %. Record the results and date. Measure your waist circumference weekly and record.

AFTER THE 4 WEEKS, SEE WHERE YOU ARE

You will be amazed by your transformation, in just 4 weeks. You will have lost at least 8 to 10 lbs., an inch or two off of your waist, a size or two in your dresses, and you will feel better than you have in years. You will sleep better, have more energy and feel a sense of accomplishment. You will finally know that with this battle plan, you can finally win the battle for life. High five your Battle Buddy, discuss going for 4 more weeks. If you decide to accept this battle plan for life you will win the war, and reclaim your health. After three months, go back to your physician and get another checkup, and blood work. Your doctor will be amazed by the results even more than you will.

CHAPTER 17:

RULES TO LIVE BY: DO'S AND DON'TS

ACCEPT THAT DISCIPLINE IS NEEDED IN YOUR LIFE TO EAT HEALTHYFOOD, LOSE WEIGHT, EXERCISE, AND TO LIFT WEIGHTS.

EAT SIX MEALS A DAY, WHEN HUNGRY, THREE MEALS, THREE SNACKS.

EAT NO FAST FOOD OF ANY KIND, EVER.

EAT NO PROCESSED FLOUR PRODUCTS, LIKE ALL BREAD, CAKES, MUFFINS, ETC. EAT ONLY WHOLE GRAIN BREAD IN SMALL AMOUNTS.

EAT NO "WESTERN DIET" FOODS: FAST FOOD, FRIED FOODS, ANIMAL FATS, RED MEAT, SATUATED FATS,

SWEETS, CHOCOLATE, SAUCES, BUTTER, OR DAIRY PRODUCTS.

EAT ONLY "HEALTHY DIET", WHOLE FOOD, VEGETABLES, FRUITS, WHOLE GRAINS, GRAIN CEREALS, BEANS, LEGUMES, FISH, BERRIES, NUTS, AND FIBER.

CUT OUT OR LIMIT ALCOHOL COMSUMPTION TO 2 OZS A DAY, PREFERABLY RED WINE.

STAY OUT OF THE SUN AND USE SFP 70 OR GREATER ON SUN EXPOSED AREAS EVERYDAY.

DO NOT SMOKE.

GET 8 HOURS OF SLEEP A NIGHT.

EXERCISE ONE HOUR A DAY, SEVEN DAYS A WEEK, ANY KIND IS ACCEPTABLE.

LIFT WEIGHTS OR ANY OTHER FORM OF RESISTANCE TRAINING 3 DAYS A WEEK.

DO NOT USE APPETITE SUPPRESSANTS, OR OVER THE COUNTER, ENERGY SHOTS OR DRINKS.

TAKE PRESCRIBED DIET DRUGS ONLY AS CLEARED AND SUPERVISED BY YOUR PHYSICIAN.

DO NOT WEIGH MORE THAN ONCE A WEEK.

TAKE EACH DAY AS IT COMES, THINK NO FURTHER THAN RIGHT NOW.

DO NOT EAT IN FRONT OF THE TV SET, EXCEPT HEALTHY SNACKS, OR LOW-FAT POP CORN.

DO NOT EAT FOR TWO HOURS BEFORE BEDTIME.

DO NOT SNACK IN THE MIDDLE OF THE NIGHT, AND IF YOU MUST, MAKE IT HEALTHY.

USE THE 20 MINUTE RULE FOR THREE MEALS A DAY.

PREPARE FOOD; DO NOT EAT OUT OF THE CAN, CARTON, PACKAGE, OR JAR.

DO NOT EAT WHEN YOU FIRST COME HOME FROM WORK.

EAT SNACKS, AND MEALS SLOWLY, SAVOR THE FOOD.

USE SMALLER PLATES TO SERVE FOOD, AND USE SMALL PORTIONS.

ONLY KEEP HEALTHY SNACKS AVAILABLE, THUS NOTHING ELSE TO TEMPT YOU.

EAT POPCORN AND NUTS ONE AT A TIME.

DRINK FLUIDS CONSTANTLY, WATER, GREEN TEA, CRYSTAL LITE, BUT NEVER SOFT DRINKS, OR CARBONATED DRINKS, EVEN ZERO CALORIE.

CHAPTER 18:

EATING RULE: THE TWENTY MINUTE RULE

"Always take a full twenty minutes to eat your first serving of food. By the clock, no second servings until a full twenty minutes have passed".

If you have recently been exposed to large masses of humanity, like when you visit a theme park, or attend a sports event, you have probably been shocked, by really seeing the epidemic of obesity in this country. It is pretty ugly to see hoards of bloated, sweating, fat parents with their over-fed children, bolting down corn dogs and nachos while searching for the funnel cake stand.

Studies of obese people have shown that they eat fast, really fast. One of my rotund friends was constantly frustrated with the food served in the upscale restaurants in France, because they served such tiny portions. Once he had stabbed the beautifully presented pate with his fork and stuffed it into his mouth in one bite, he had nothing to do until the next course arrived. So he complained, and ate all of the bread on the table and asked the other guests "are you going to eat that bread?" He did not savor the food or take a healthy, civilized amount of time to eat it.

We have all been guilty of eating too fast. We are in a rush, or during family meals, competing with ravenous teenagers, who might get that last salmon filet if we don't hurry. Dinners in our family with the kids were more akin to a shark feeding frenzy than a civilized ritual. Do you find yourself loading up your second plate at a buffet brunch within the first 10 or 15 minutes of finishing the first?

Low blood sugar levels and an empty stomach are two known stimuli to appetite. Most of the time low blood sugar levels are corrected within minutes of eating in normal people. Even when insulin and glucose levels return to normal, there is still a sense of hunger.

We have known for years that there is a satiety center in the brain that turns on about twenty minutes after beginning to eat. Removal of the satiety center of the brain in rats has resulted in sumo-like rats the size of small dogs. A small protein called leptin produced in the white adipocytes (fat cells) found in the stomach and intestines, is the major substance that signals that part of the brain that you are full. It has its full effect around 20 minutes after beginning to eat.

This observation led to the "twenty minute rule" for our family dinners. The rule is simple, and it works. Each diner is allowed a single modest first serving of the dinner. Serve actual real portions (small) on smaller plates with about half of what you would normally eat. As we begin the meal, a silent 20 minute timer is started. Nobody is allowed a second serving until the full twenty minutes have elapsed. Children, of course, hate this rule, and will tell you that it is inhumane, that they will starve to death, and that they are going to call child protective services because they are being tortured.

When you implement this rule, you too will have to sit there 20 minutes anyway, so you might as well eat slowly, and with nothing else to do for the twenty minutes, you might even risk entering into a conversation with other members of the family. You may be shocked to hear more than the usual indistinct monotone grunts from your teenagers, and may actually have a semi-normal conversation. You will no longer have anxiety about the remaining food being gobbled up, and you will rarely want seconds. Neither will the kids.

If you are dining with your spouse, your Battle Buddy, you should still implement the rule. It takes away the rushed, frantic feeling meals can have, and allows for conversation. Even when by yourself, use the rule. The experts say not to read when you eat, but when eating alone, we find it helps pass the time, and help us make the full twenty minutes.

Try it. You have nothing to lose but the anxiety and the weight.

CHAPTER 19:

TOGETHER: DOING IT AS A COUPLE, BATTLE BUDDIES

IF THERE ARE TWO OF YOU

If you live with someone in a domestic relationship you need their support, or better, their participation to truly adapt this life-saving, life-sustaining, life-style. It very difficult to go it alone, living with a domestic partner who brings home chocolate chip cookies, or continues to make homemade bread.

If you have been living together for more than 10 years, then the chances are overwhelming that you both have fallen prey to an insidious 5 to 10 pound weight gain a year. Since almost 70% of older adults are overweight or obese, you are probably one of those couples. Gayne and I certainly were.

By checking your individual BMI's, and waist circumference and factoring in any known risk factors for

ASCVD, and any already emerging problems like "borderline" hypertension, a bad lipid profile or diabetes, it will be apparent that you are both at risk for early death, and a life of miserable disability. Who is going first, and who is going to take care of whom? That's what got our attention.

We want to live to see our grandchildren grow up; to remain independent, functional, vital, energetic, and mobile. There are no short cuts. The only way to get there, and stay there, is to change what you weigh, what you eat, and to add regular exercise and resistance training to your routine.

If you could prevent your domestic partner from developing pancreatic cancer, wouldn't you make the effort? If they have increasing weight gain, especially with a BMI greater than 30, a male with a waist 40 inches or greater, or a female with a waist of 36 inches or greater, they have a diagnosis as bad as cancer, because they are going to die sooner than they should, and with great suffering and disability. As Battle Buddies, aren't you supposed to watch each other's back and keep each other out of harm's way?

Together, read and discuss the horrific statistics, curtailed longevity and the growing list of diseases linked to overweight and obesity (now more than 38). Recognize that you have accepted the specious mantra of, "I'm getting older, and being heavier is part of it, so I might as well accept it". If you really believe that "graceful aging" is accepting and resigning yourself to poor health, then you have surrendered and lost the battle, without a fight. You have been led to believe that your abdominal fat, hypertension, diabetes, and all the other ensuing diseases are just part of aging, or that they "run in the family". Nothing could be further from the truth.

You have been told to "age gracefully", accept yourself as you are, and to slow down. If you accept this philosophy, you will slow down, alright, and will become sedentary, older than your years, and will become a sick invalid.

By this time you have probably fallen into the Middle Age Couple Obesity syndrome (MACOS). MACOS is characterized by no sex life; eating in front of the TV or in bed. You are watching yourself and your partner continue to gain weight, become more depressed, and losing your enthusiasm for living, and your relationship.

Fecundity, the ability to be "fruitful", or to get pregnant and have children is inversely related to the couple's body weight. This means, the heavier the man and woman trying to reproduce, the less chance of the woman has of becoming pregnant and having a child. Such a couple is termed "subfecund". In one of many studies on the subject, it was suggested that a major part of the problem is lack of trying. Really? Perhaps MACOS has crept into the relationship.

The nurturer of the couple, usually the wife, will have to take the initiative. In my experience in the ER, it's always the wife who nags the old boy into coming in. Wives save thousands of husbands' lives each year by insisting they be evaluated for "little problems", like passing blood in their stool or an elephant on their chest. That is the major reason that married men live about 8 years longer than unmarried men. The nurturer of the couple will have to "sell" or mandate the life-style change to their partner.

It is probably impossible to truly change your diet and life-style without your partner fully committed. For example, how do you keep your living space free of lethal foods if your partner is frying up some pork chops, or bringing home pizza? I cannot resist ice cream if it is accessible. Since you are going to fight the battle to save your health and gain functional longevity, you need a complicit spouse, a Battle Buddy by your side.

My college aged son came home to visit and brought his favorite ice cream, coffee. When he returned to school, some of the ice cream was left in our freezer. I told Gayne that I would throw it away, so that we wouldn't be tempted to eat it. As her Battle Buddy, I was getting rid of the lethal food to protect us both from succumbing. Of course, the second she wasn't looking, I ate it directly out of the carton, and then licked inside of the carton, until a forensic expert from CSI could not have detected a micro trace of coffee ice cream in that container. Why? Because it was there. When Gayne next saw me, she immediately asked, "You ate the ice cream didn't you Bob?" I thought it was a heroic action, kind of like jumping on the live hand grenade to save my Battle Buddy.

If your partner is heavy and does not want to participate, it will be much more difficult for you to adopt THE BATTLE BUDDY DIET program by yourself. If you do it alone and succeed, you will begin to look much better than your partner, and will begin getting attention from others. In my limited experience, if one partner truly changes what they eat and how they look, while the other continues remain overweight, the relationship will become seriously strained.

If you both want to change, commit together, become sworn Battle Buddies for the 30 days, and go for it with mutual support. We think it is a good idea for the two of you to shop together for food for the first couple of trips. Check food nutrition labels together, pick out vegetables and fruits that you both like, and monitor each other to keep lethal foods out of the basket. Battle Buddies keep each other out of trouble and away from harmful temptations. Go through the house together and remove all the lethal foods, and give them away. You cannot keep chips, processed snacks or sweets for visiting "guests", you will eat them.

If the two of you are honest with yourselves, and stick to **THE BATTLE BUDDY DIET** program for 30 days, the changes will be dramatic. You will lose around 8 pounds or more and reshape your body. You will have fewer chronic pains and inflammation, more energy, less depression and more body image esteem. Your sex life will start to be rekindled and your blood pressure, lipids and glucose metabolism will all improve.

Once on the program, permanently, your weight will become optimal, and most of the physiologic consequences of obesity will disappear. Most people on the program will be able to stop their hypertension, diabetic and lipid medicines. Repair of the endothelium of your arteries will start naturally and you will slow aging.

Once Gayne and I made it 30 days, we were so shocked and pleased with our results, that we kept ourselves on the program until we both reached our optimal BMI's, and took 6 to 8 inches off of our waists. We both reached our ideal weight, and most likely that is what you weighed in High School. Today, we have continued the same diet but with more healthy calories since we are maintaining our weight and not trying to lose anymore.

This Battle Buddy thing with your spouse is a good thing for more than just supporting each other in our life-style change. Knowing that you have someone who would lay down their life for you and puts you before themselves is the secret to a real relationship. We feel closer and more attracted to each other. I think our mutual project of investigating the medical literature together, developing our own diet and healthy life-style plan and applying to our own lives, brought us closer together. Having success has helped revive our relationship. We have a few suggested rules for couples that undertake the program together. You may think of some of your own.

BATTLE BUDDY RULES

You may not comment on your Battle Buddy's weight, except when asked, and then you may only use positive comments, like: "I can really see a difference in your hips, they look much better".

You may never comment on what your Battle Buddy is eating or drinking. Only they are responsible for their own mouth and what goes in it. Do not police them or "take their inventory".

When asked the inevitable, "Do these pants make me look fat?" Remember only positive comments, like "They look so much better on you now, your butt is getting smaller."

If you are making a healthy snack, like fruit, or raw carrots and broccoli, dipped in a low calorie, no fat dressing, make some for your Battle Buddy.

You should share the responsibility of making healthy meals, and you are not allowed to be critical of the other's efforts.

You may reveal your weight to your Battle Buddy only if you chose to do so, but you should never be asked.

Make a point of encouraging each other, with at least two positive comments a day, like "You are looking so much younger", because you will!

Nag, blackmail, bribe or threaten to get your Battle Buddy to have regular diagnostic tests and appropriate blood work. Make sure your Battle Buddy has a colonoscopy at age 50.

If you have a compulsive eating disorder, or deep psychological wounds that cause you to eat too much of the wrong foods and you cannot control it, get professional help.

CHAPTER 20:

SAVE YOUR CHILDREN: THE FAMILY BATTLE PLAN

OBESITY AND DISEASE IN CHILDREN

You can see it for yourself. Everywhere you look, you see more and more overweight, obese kids. The statistics are scary. In 1980 only 6.5% of kids were considered obese. By 2008 that number had tripled to 20%, and now is passing 30%. This is a legitimate epidemic. This generation of children will be the first in history to have a shorter life expectancy than their parents.

Elementary aged kids are developing type II diabetes, hyperlipidemia, fatty liver disease, hypertension, sleep apnea and premature puberty. The onset of puberty is triggered by body weight. Typically, when a female reaches a weight of around 96-100 lbs. they will experience their first menses. It is very scary for me to see 6 and 7year old girls developing breasts, pubic hair and having periods. By the way, it' not the hormones in the food, it's their body weight.

Increasingly, I see 6 to 12year old children in my practice that are on oral diabetic medications, statins and hypertensive medications. In my medical training, I avoided pediatrics because I could not emotionally cope with innocent children developing leukemia, brain tumors or other cancers. Just being in the presence of a little child, bald from the latest round of chemotherapy, heroic and full of optimism, fighting their cancer, would make me weep. Now I see the overweight and obese kids and teenagers with the same prognosis, like the pediatric cancer victims, their lives will be afflicted with horrible suffering and premature deaths.

Teenagers in the United States and other developed countries now have full blown ASCVD. Coronary artery bypass and stent operations are now being performed on 15 year old patients. The incidences of obesity linked diseases are becoming common place in kids and teenagers. Previously rare diseases in teenagers, like: cholecystitis, fatty liver, sleep apnea, GERD, pulmonary hypertension, cardiomyopathy, myocardial infarction, accelerated osteoarthritis, depression, eating disorders, low self-esteem, and obesity linked cancers are becoming all too common.

WHY? AND HOW DID THIS HAPPEN?

Theories abound about how our generation of children got so fat. The simplest explanations are the same ones that have made their Baby Boomer parents overweight and obese; the Western Diet. Too many of the wrong foods and lack of physical activity are central to the problem. Certainly, high sugar, high fat, and processed foods in abundance are the toxins that have fueled the childhood obesity epidemic. Ready access, relentless marketing, by the food industry and the unknowing co-conspirators, the parents, are all to blame.

Multiple studies of childhood obesity have consistently shown that there is a direct correlation of television and videogame hours with the expanding waist and decreasing athletic ability in small children and teenagers. Even in 1 year to 6 year old kids, their waist size significantly increased directly related to more hours of television watching. Children who do not sit down to dinner with the family are significantly heavier than those that do. Just like their parents, kids who eat in front of the television are heavier. While raising our children, we never allowed television or video games during the school week, even in the summertime. Our kids were allowed and encouraged to read during the week, and shocked us by doing so.

Fat parents have fat children. Sorry, Honey Boo Boo. If the wrong foods are all around them, like candy, chips, sugary sodas, fruit juices, mammalian meat, and a plethora of ubiquitous processed foods, and Mom and Dad are eating them, so will their kids. I don't know many 4 year olds who shop for food, though many of them lobby for harmful foods while their parents shop. Ignorant or un-caring parents are to blame, at least in early childhood.

Teenaged obesity is a consequence of childhood obesity. An overweight child will become and overweight or obese teenager, and adult, with very few exceptions. Reversing the epidemic of teenaged obesity may be impossible, without radical changes in the marketing of unhealthy foods.

My own kids went to an up-scale public high school, in an affluent neighborhood. Their lunch choices were limited to the vendors on campus: Taco Bell, Pizza Hut, and Burger King. Soft drink and snack machines were available all day long, dispensing very unhealthy fare any time they wanted it. It was not considered "hip" to bring your own lunch, or to eat healthy foods. In those days, kids that ate fresh whole foods were considered weird, or Vegan.

Instead of celebrities asking if we "Have milk?", or touting "Beef, it's what's for dinner", perhaps we need a few enlightened ones to suggest a whole food salad, fresh fruit, or filet of wild salmon. If it becomes the "in thing" to eat healthy whole foods, a prudent diet, the problem can be mitigated. Making good tasting healthy foods available at schools, from grade school through high school is the other part of the solution. Michelle Obama you are right, but you realize what you are up against.

PARENTS' RESPONSIBILITY

I do not know any parents who would knowingly harm their children. I know of none who would knowingly poison their children, and cripple or disable them for life. Yet, that is exactly what is happening in the majority of American families. If you are feeding your children the lethal Western Diet, you are causing disease and starting your progeny down a lifelong path of suffering, illness and premature death. Even if they do not become overweight or obese, the wrong foods will damage them and cause preventable diseases and cancers. ASCVD is found in autopsies of American 2 year olds on the Western Diet.

Allowing morbid obesity in children has been legally considered a form of child abuse or child neglect in an increasing number of cases. Parents must step up and start infants and toddlers on the whole food, prudent diet from the start. If your kids are older, it is not too late. If they see their parents change what they eat, and see them exercise; they will most likely follow suit.

If your children are older, explain that the changes that your family is making in their diet are for just 4 weeks. Let them express their feelings about the change. Yes, they will call you cruel, weird and uncaring…even bad parents. You will be told that you are not like the other "really nice parents" of their friends. Exactly; you're not. You will not allow them to eat "heart attack pills", the lethal foods that cause them grave harm. Try to get them to buy into the family battle plan, a 4 week experiment of changing the diet of all of the family because it better. Challenge them to stay the course and earn the right to be Battle Buddies.

With our own children, we implemented THE BATTLE BUDDY DIET program, when they were teenagers. They thought the idea was "lame" and they easily found ways to cheat. After all, lethal food is everywhere and easy to get. They snuck sodas, chips and burgers outside of the house. We did not try to police them, rather just kept the rules for food and meals in the house consistent. There were no lethal foods allowed in the home, and they grudgingly agreed to abide by that rule.

Over a period of the four weeks, they stopped cheating and started to reluctantly embrace the whole foods prudent diet. They even admitted that they felt more energy and seemed to perform better on their sports teams. Today, as young adults, they still eat a whole foods prudent diet, exercise and do resistance training. However, even now, my son and I have been known to stop at the "IN-AND-OUT BURGER" and enjoy a lethal burger and maybe a lethal serving of fries. None of us have to be perfect, just consistent. Studies show that children will adopt the diet of their parents, as adults in the majority of cases.

Children have a right to healthy nutrition, just as they have the right to be cared for and protected by their parents. Do the right thing, not the easy thing. It will pay dividends for you and your children.

THE BATTLE BUDDY DIET, KID STYLE: TIPS

Empty the house of all "bad "foods. Kids cannot eat it if it is not available, and they will eat it if it is there. Do not hoard your own secret bad food somewhere, they will find it and eat it. You lose your food and your credibility.

Five meals a day: Breakfast, Lunch, Dinner and two healthy snacks. No other eating.

Eat scheduled dinner as a family, or at least as many as can be assembled. Use the twenty minute rule. You may only eat what if offered.

Close the kitchen after dinner. No refrigerator grazing or snack seeking after the evening meal. No food is allowed to be stored anywhere but the kitchen.

No eating in your room or in front of the TV or while playing video games.

No fruit juice, especially for infants and toddlers, the sugar content is criminal, the same or greater than a sugared soda!

No cow's milk, ever. Get them to like almond milk or soy milk. Growing children do not need cow's milk for calcium or protein. Fortified soy or almond milk is better, and protein can come from beans, and fish.

Do not sell this diet as a "diet". This is how we eat, for life, and the way we think you should eat the rest of your life. They will do what they see you do, not what you tell them to do.

No fast food, especially as a reward. Baked "sweet potato fries" are healthy and just as good tasting as the lethal fast food French fries (hold the catsup).

No special meals; you should never be a short order cook. They must eat what is served. Let them help make the healthy menu choices, and even help prepare it.

Serve meals on plates, not buffet style. Use smaller plates, with small servings.

Bring healthy snacks on car trips, or buy them at the grocery store along the way, in lieu of the fast food places.

Never have different eating rules for different kids, "You can't have the buttered popcorn since you are on a diet, but your skinny sister can". That creates two eating disorders with one thoughtless statement.

Never comment on how much they eat or don't eat. NEVER, NEVER, NEVER, comment on their weight, or figure.

Allow indiscretions in diet at parties or during special celebrations. Of course they can have some of the ice cream and cake at the Birthday party, or other bad foods on special Holidays, like pumpkin pie at Thanksgiving.

Let them help pack their lunches for school with healthy choices, unless there are truly healthy choices available on the school menu. Some elementary schools now have healthy food sections and will make sure your small child picks only from that section.

Do not punish kids for not cleaning their plates. They will eat what they need; just don't be blackmailed into giving them alternative choices; this is what's for dinner, eat it or leave it (after twenty minutes). Likewise, don't reward them for eating.

No social media, of any kind, at any meal. No cell phone, I pad, music systems, or ear buds of any kind. Implement the same rule with visiting relatives or guests during a meal.

It is good to make eating new foods, especially vegetables, a game for infants and toddlers. "Look at the broccoli trees; let's bite the tops off, like Daddy does!" "Batman eats beets to make himself so strong".

Insist that your kids have a regular after school sport, from early age through high school. It does not have to be starting for the varsity; a club sport will do nicely. It burns calories, exhausts them, keeps them in shape, helps friendships, self-esteem and keeps them busy.

Do not label foods "good" or "bad", rather refer to them as "healthy" or "unhealthy".

When they are older, take them food shopping. Let them select the healthy foods of their choice. Teach them to read ingredients on food labels, so they can learn to make healthy choices.

Beware of the cereals they crave. Always check the sugar content. The average American 4 year old eats 17 teaspoons of sugar a day, and they don't buy it themselves.

When you take them out to eat, teach them to order off of the menu, to substitute more vegetables for fries, and to bake instead of fry the fish.

Use Splenda as a sugar substitute. It has never been shown to cause cancer or disease; sugar has.

Do not comment on the unhealthy diets of their friends. They may eat what their parents allow them to eat. We just think that some of the foods that others eat are unhealthy for you and our family.

CHAPTER 21:

EATING TIPS

GET RID OF ALL THE LETHAL FOODS: The one of the first steps in starting a real life-style diet change is to get rid of all of the bad foods in your home, at work and in the car. Load up all of the chips, low fat muffins, fat free cookies and even your secret stash of snickers. Take them to work, put them out in the break room and watch them evaporate.

EAT FIVE OR MORE TIMES A DAY: Small amounts of only the healthy foods, like berries or limited nuts as a between meal snacks. Carry your baby carrots or berries in the car with you.

EAT BREAKFAST EVERY DAY, NO EXCEPTIONS: Breakfast is the meal most likely meal to be fully metabolized during the day. The right amount of protein, grain and fat free dairy, or soy will fill you up and prevent the 10:30 am, "I'm starving!" syndrome.

DO NOT EAT IF YOU DON'T FEEL HUNGRY: If you are with someone else who is eating, have a cup of green tea or water and save your healthy meal or snack for when you really want it.

SAVOR YOUR FOOD AND EAT IT SLOWLY: You should really enjoy the taste of the food, pause between bites, and apply the "twenty minute" rule to all meals.

IN THE BEGINNING :KEEP AN HONEST LOG OF EVERYTHING YOU EAT: It is frequently shocking how much "phantom" food we eat, like the two donut holes in the break area at work, that really didn't count because we didn't eat one of the jelly donuts. In the early part of this program, you should track all that you eat, to insure that you are not eating phantom "lethal foods".

TAKE HEALTHY SNACKS WITH YOU: Great for when you are in traffic, movie theaters, concerts, traveling or on an airplane, take them along with you when you study. Fresh fruit, dried fruits, dry whole grain cereals, raw vegetables or a limited number of nuts in a take-along zip lock bag, are all healthy snacks.

DRINK AT LEAST 10oz OF FLUID EACH TIME YOU EAT: It is filling and will help extend the satiety provided by the healthy foods. Soups that are animal fat free, like fresh vegetable soup, are healthy and more filling.

DO NOT EAT MEALS IN FRONT OF THE TV SET: You will not appreciate what you are eating, you will eat faster, and you will eat more. If you are watching a family movie together, have low fat microwave popcorn, or vegetable snacks, or dried fruits.

NEVER EAT IN THE BED: The bed should be for only two things; sleeping and sex. If there is a TV or computer in your bedroom, and you eat in bed, your relationship is in serious decline and if you are a couple, you are probably in the "MACOS" rut.

IF YOU DRIVE A LOT, OR ON CAR TRIPS, DO NOT STOP AT THE FAST FOOD, OR TRUCKSTOP PLACES: It is far better to pull off of the freeway into a small town, find the grocery store, or Mom and Pop convenience store. They have fresh fruit, dried fruits, salad bars and vegetables. If healthy food is all that is available in the car, that is all that can get eaten.

WHEN DINING OUT, DO NOT ALLOW THE BREAD AND CHIPS TO BE PUT ON THE TABLE: Always pick the fresh fish over animal meat. If a healthy entrée is served on pasta, ask if it can be served on brown rice, or in lieu of the pasta, could you have extra fresh vegetables? Hold the fries, if they reach the table, they will be eaten. Always have salad dressing on the side; olive oil and balsamic vinegar are always a better alternative for creamy, high fat dressings.

WHEN DINING OUT, SPLIT A MEAL: Portions in most restaurants are massive. Splitting a main entrée on to smaller plates, with extra vegetables, eaten slowly, is plenty filling. If some is left, take it home. If you simply must have some of the dessert, like the Mud Pie, order one for the entire table and pass it around. Then take only two small bites!

FORGET THE MIDNIGHT SNACK: I used to love to get up at around 3 am and eat ice cream right out of the carton. I have learned to get up, in the dark, and have a glass of water and go back to bed. You should do the same. Do not go to the kitchen after hours.

DO NOT EAT RIGHT BEFORE BED: It's not just the fact that the calories consumed will be metabolized slower during sleep, they will more likely be stored as fat. Furthermore, eating right before bed disturbs sleep, critical to a healthy lifestyle.

NEVER EAT DIRECTLY OUT OF A CAN, JAR OR CARTON: The French got this right. It always pays to take time to prepare, and serve a meal or snack, even just for you. Do not snack on the food as you prepare it, it is far better to have some carrots on the side, or fluids.

DO NOT GO STRAIGHT TO THE REFRIGERATOR WHEN YOU GET HOME FROM WORK: This is a lethal habit. After an ER shift, I used to throw down my briefcase on the kitchen counter, open the refrigerator and start eating. I would eat quickly, and a lot. Grab an apple or plum if you must, then go put up your briefcase, check the mail, change clothes and then plan and prepare the meal.

USE SMALL PLATES AND SMALL SERVING: It has been shown in multiple studies that people will eat less food on smaller plates and be just as satisfied as eating much larger servings. Again, eating slowly is the key.

DO NOT EAT FAST FOOD AFTER A NIGHT OF PARTYING: After drinking party quantities of alcohol, many people get hungry, and someone always has the idea to order pizza or drive to local fast food joint. Alcohol stimulates appetite, and is caloric. In fact, alcohol is about 7 calories per gram, and will always be metabolized first, since it cannot be stored as glycogen or fat. However, those extra calories from the burgers or tacos you ate, after drinking the alcohol, can and will be stored as fat.

READ THE NUTRITION LABEL ON EVERYTHING BEFORE YOU BUY IT: Put your reading glasses on in the food store, sellers make the nutritional material intentionally printed in a microscopic font. Be sure to check serving size, sometimes the identical products will change serving size to make the calories appear fewer. If the label says "Trans-fats", or "hydrogenated" anything, or has significant saturated fats > 1gram, or carbohydrates > 40grams, or sugar >10 grams, do not buy it.

DO NOT BUY OR EAT ANYTHING THAT IS PROCESSED: Man made snacks, like potato chips, cookies, cakes, and even fruit rolls are loaded with lethal substances. When in doubt, eat only natural foods "whole foods" and you will never go wrong. Any food or drink made or manipulated by man, is universally unhealthy.

BE CAREFUL WITH ENERGY BARS, DRINKS AND MEAL REPLACEMENTS: Most "healthy energy bars" are really just candy bars. Limit yourself to those high in protein and low in fat, carbohydrates and sugar. Some can be useful as a source of complete healthy protein with relatively few calories, but beware of added sugars, milk protein, milk chocolate, high calorie fruits and excessive nuts.

USE SUGAR REPLACEMENTS: There has never been credible evidence that these substances harm man. The three major types are all acceptable and can be used to sweeten cereal, in cooking and to sweeten drinks. I personally use "Splenda" or sucralose; it tastes good and is used the same way as sugar on cereal or in cooking, and is absolutely not associated with any cancer risk.

USE COOKING OILS SPARINGLY: Limit use to olive oil or canola and use as little as possible. Use small amounts to sear fresh vegetables, and then stir "fry" on high heat, using water to continue cooking. Cooked mushrooms make their own sauce supplying "healthy gravy" for multiple vegetable meals.

USE SPICES AND VARIETY OF FOODS: Spices can make bland food good and should be experimented with in healthy food preparation. Try a new vegetable like an exotic squash, or a new type of mushroom. There are some great tasting healthy receipts available on the internet, and in books of healthy "whole food" diets.

AT THE PARTY, STICK TO THE HEALTHY FOODS: You will most likely find yourself competing for the big shrimp, and fresh salmon and vegetable tray with other thin, attractive people. The overweight guests will be inhaling chicken wings, spearing the little meatballs, spreading the Brie, or inhaling super nachos with extra guacamole.

DRINK TEA INSTEAD OF COFFEE: Well, ok, you can have one big cup of coffee in the morning, but then make it tea. Coffee and tea both have positive health benefits, but green tea may be a magic elixir of youth. It has amazing substances that fight cancer, lower blood pressure, decrease diabetes, improve blood lipids, increase longevity and it increases metabolism. The increased metabolism significantly accelerates weight loss in matched dieters. Regular tea is cured green tea, and is almost as good.

DO NOT EAT CANDY OR SWEETS: For the sake of the women of the world, there must be some tolerance of chocolate. In fact, dark chocolate, not milk chocolate, has been shown to provide some antioxidants and improve mood. Milk chocolate is a lethal food. Try to stick only to the dark type, without other lethal ingredients. It counts for calories! A good alternative is to cut up a dark chocolate healthy protein bar and eat the pieces slowly like candy. No pastries, cheese cake, cakes, muffins, crème Brule, baked Alaska, or any of those great tasting desserts. Fresh fruit, berries, non-fat sugar free yogurt, mixed with a little sprinkled Splenda is a great tasting alternative.

CHAPTER 22:

EXERCISE: THE BATTLE PLAN'S CRITICAL ELEMENT

WAIT, THERE IS A MAGIC PILL!

If I told you there is a pill, taken daily, that has absolutely been proven by the world-wide scientific community to do the following: help reduce your weight and keep it off, significantly decrease your chances of getting multiple types of cancer, stroke, heart attack, diabetes, high blood pressure and some thirty other nasty debilitating diseases, wouldn't you want this pill? This miraculous pill will even make you look and feel younger, eradicate depression, increase brain function, decrease senile dementia, improve all of your blood lipids and inflammatory markers, insure mental and functional independence with aging, relive stress, preserve muscle mass, increase longevity, and will literally reverse aging, by making your physiologic age (body age) younger than your chronological age and even jump-start your waning sex life!

Would you want such a pill? Let's call it the "H-pill" for healthy. It has no serious side effects, and can be taken by everyone, at any age. What if you had to vigorously (at 65% of maximum capacity) exercise for one hour each day and lift weights 30 minutes three times a week, to get the H-pill? Would you do it? The H-pill is frequently prescribed, but cannot be purchased at any price.

All of us would want the H-pill, and maybe even agree to prioritize and complete the required exercise to get the pill; after all, what do you have if you don't have your health? Don't we all want to look our best and maintain an independent, functional life-style? Sadly, only about one in ten of you will actually decide to earn the H-pill, and commit to the required exercise. That is the percentage of adult Americans that exercise vigorously on a regular basis (8-12%). Of course, the irony is that the H-pill is available to all of us, since the H-pill is the exercise.

Some 50% of us do some type of exercise on sporadic basis, which will not qualify you for the proven healthy benefits of the H-pill. Finally, some 25% of you do no exercise of any kind, ever. A sedentary life style is a huge independent risk factor for developing all of the nasty diseases associated with obesity, especially ASCVD, heart attack, stroke and dangerous blood clots of the legs. Sedentary people do not survive as long as others with known ASCVD risk factors, like smoking, who exercise.

That's right! A smoker, who exercises regularly, will last longer, and maintain more function, than a sedentary person that does not smoke. These totally sedentary, akinetic people really need the H-pill, "STAT", as we say in the business.

THE BATTLE BUDDY DIET AND EXERCISE

Without one hour of vigorous exercise a day, seven days a week, and thirty minutes of weight training, three times a week, you cannot truly adapt an optimal, healthy life-style. Remember, our mission is to reach a healthy weight and stay there, while maintaining a high level of function and independence. This goal cannot be attained, or maintained without a full dose of the required H-pill, the exercise.

The food recommended in this program is the healthiest diet "for life", that the two of us could find, after searching all of the credible scientific and medical literature. Eating the right foods, and avoiding the "lethal foods", with calorie restriction, will result in a predictable weight loss, improvement in blood lipids, blood pressure, will decrease the development of diabetes (II) and will significantly increase longevity. However, without the H-pill, the exercise and resistance training, you can undo many of the benefits of your better diet and still risk loss of functional independence.

It is well documented that men and women loose muscle mass with age. In men it is about 7 pounds per decade after the age of 30, unless they regularly exercise and "stress" the muscles. More alarming is the fact that loss of the muscle mass from disuse, further results in loss of neural connections with aging, which means the atrophied muscle, will no longer respond to training, and is not functional thereafter. This muscle is lost forever! This same type of muscle loss has been documented in females with dieting and aging. Do we really want to have to order one of those "push up seats" for our recliners, when we cannot get out of a chair or off of the toilet without help?

DIET AND MUSCLE MASS

Our program is not a simple calorie restricted diet to follow for a few weeks, then go back to your old diet, resolved to "eat less". No popular, "fad" diet has ever been shown to keep the lost weight off. These ineffectual strategies include: the packaged food diets, delivered prepared food diets, meal substitute diets, and using drinks or "nutrition" bars. They will not last long term unless they are all that you eat for the rest of your life. You must permanently change what you eat and exercise to maintain weight loss and your health.

Fad or crash diets frequently ignore the critical maintenance of muscle mass while reducing weight. Some 30% of weight lost in most diets, is pure muscle! That means that a 20 pound weight loss would mean a loss of 6 pounds of muscle. We all need all of the functional, trained muscle mass we can get, as we age.

Maintenance of muscle mass requires only two basics: (1) exercise and stress (resistance training) and (2) protein, with essential amino acids. Our program advocates both as part of a permanent life style change. This strategy is not "body building"; it is to insure that functional, strong, responsive muscle is there when you need it, for the remainder of your life.

ADVANTAGES OF MUSCLE MASS MAINTENANCE

Besides the obvious advantage of having muscle to function, there are other important metabolic advantages of maintaining and increasing muscle mass. Muscle at rest, burns calories five to seven times faster than other body tissues, and while exercising muscle metabolism increases a staggering 15 to 25 times greater than other body tissues. It takes more energy to metabolize protein, the major building blocks of muscle, than for metabolizing fat or carbohydrates. Each pound of muscle in your body will burn an extra 30 to 50 calories a day.

Most weight control exercise programs recommend anaerobic type exercises, like running and walking, to maximize calorie burning. We now know that vigorous resistance training for an hour burns almost the same calories as running at 70% effort for an hour! Vigorous anaerobic exercise increases body metabolic rate for 8 to 10 hours after the exertion. Resistance training, (weight lifting) is better: recent studies have shown a surprising 48 hours of increased metabolism after weight/resistance training!

Exercise and maintenance of well-toned muscle mass, with optimal body weight, is an attainable "fountain of youth". Compared to others their age, people who maintain optimal weight and exercise on a regular basis, look younger, feel younger, more energetic, and independent. They are much more likely to maintain their intellectual capacity, have less illness, fewer injuries, an active sex life, and not surprisingly, are much more likely to describe their lives as "happy".

People who maintain, or increase their muscle mass can eat more calories than those who have less muscle. That is the major reason that men can generally eat more calories for weight loss or weight maintenance than women. By maintaining muscle or building muscle you can eat more food and keep an optimal body weight.

EXERCISE, HEALTH, LONGEVITY

I had a physician friend during my medical training. He was a top-drawer cardiologist. I keep using the past tense because he is deceased. He had a standing joke. Every time he would spot me going out for a run at lunch time, or after work, he would smile and say, "That heart of yours only has so many beats in a lifetime, and you are wasting yours running up hills!" He was not overweight but never exercised. Sadly, he died of a massive heart attack at the age of 46.

What my cardiologist friend did not know is that exactly the opposite is true. The more consistently and vigorously you exercise the longer you will live. Walking vigorously only an average of thirty minutes a day has been shown to prevent weight gain, and decreases the incidence of lethal abdominal obesity. Doing the required one hour a day will give you your best chance for maintenance or weight, health and high quality longevity.

There have been hundreds of studies and many thousands of patients followed for thirty to forty years or more, to investigate the reasons some live longer, with less disease than others. Central to all of the observations and factors, is the fact that regular exercise decreases your chances of being dangerously overweight, of acquiring metabolic syndrome, of developing ASCVD and of dying prematurely.

It has been shown time and time again, that regular exercise will change serum lipids for the better, by decreasing the LDL's (bad lipids) and increasing the HDL's (good lipids), lower blood pressure, and decrease insulin resistance (early diabetes), all risk factors for ASCVD. Resistance training has been shown to do the same, and both activities seem to greatly decrease intravascular inflammation, the key to ASCVD and unstable plaques leading to stroke and heart attack.

The risk for many cancers is greatly reduced by regular exercise; particularly prostate cancer in men and possibly ovarian cancer in women. Walking only a mile a day has been shown to protect older women's risk of dying of ASCVD by 50%. There is exciting new evidence that physical exercise increases and maintains intellectual function. Exercise is critical to the repair and new growth of neurons in the brain and nervous system. Some 90% of the successful participants in the National Weight Control Registry, who lost a mean of 66 lbs. and kept if off for at least five years, exercise regularly and consistently eat a healthy diet.

The lucky older people who exercise regularly are more likely to describe their lives as "happy" and suffer less depression, than those that do not exercise. Levels of testosterone increase in both sexes during vigorous exercise and resistance training, so it is not surprising that most men and women who regularly work out have more sex and would describe their sex lives as "good" or "satisfying".

Another proven benefit of exercise is a reduction in falls, accidents and less absenteeism at work. The combination of regular endurance training, resistance training, and exercises for flexibility and balance produce highly functional individuals capable of self-care, high self-esteem, and a sense of independence. They look good, feel good, and will live to see their grandchildren grow up.

Earn the magic H-pill, buy paying the dues. It is one of the single best investments you can make in your health, even if you don't lose weight and continue your bad eating habits. Regular exercise alone will help you live longer and healthier. It is incredible to understand that the leading cause of death in the USA, obesity/diet induced ASCVD, is preventable, and even reversible with proper food and exercise.

Body builders have a pretty basic pragmatic saying, "Eat right, work out, sleep". In my case, I don't live to work out. I work out to live.

CHAPTER 23:

STARTING REGULAR EXERCISE

HOW TO START AND MAKE IT A PRIORITY

Very few people need a doctor's approval to begin an exercise program. Obviously, if you have a chronic medical problem, like a past history of heart disease or any other chronic disease currently causing disability, check with your physician before starting. Otherwise, jump right in. No matter what your weight, blood pressure or lipid status, exercise will improve your health.

"But I hate exercise, it's painful". Quit whining and accept the fact that it must be part of a healthy life-style, and is an essential ingredient in this program. Take control and inject some good old fashioned discipline back into your life. You must first prioritize to always schedule exercise on a daily basis. I know you have an abundance of reasons you cannot commit to a regular schedule. I have heard them all and used most of them myself for the last few years.

Get up earlier, walk at lunch, walk after work, walk the dog, take the stairs, park further from the front door at work, run the back stairs of the hotel with the pitiful gym, do some push-ups and dips while you watch TV, join a gym, work in the garden, take an exercise or cycling class, ride a bike, walk on an elliptical machine, ski, surf, snowboard, play tennis, basketball, swim, run, etc. Don't just sit there in your "sports chair" watching the kids practice soccer, run around the field yourself for a while, or help the coach and do the drills, chase some balls. You can exercise in your hotel room on the road, or even while sitting on a plane.

YES, AN HOUR A DAY

Remember, the total time of exercise should be an hour a day, but that does not mean it has to all be done at once. If you can squeeze in 30 minutes of walking at lunch, you can later ride a bike for the remaining thirty minutes. Other activities count, like working in the garden, doing house work, dancing and even vigorous sex. Keep a daily record of your exercise in your day timer or on your phone. There are simple, free applications available for your I-phone or android that can help you calculate the approximate calories burned, by almost any type of exercise.

While on this diet, limiting your calories to 500 below daily requirements will result in a total of 3500 of your excessive calories being "burned" a week, or one pound of weight loss a week. In addition, if you walked for 60 minutes a day (about 3.5 miles) you would burn an additional 450 to 500 calories a day, increasing your weight loss to almost two pounds a week, or around 24-30 pounds in this 12 week program.

To benefit from exercise, you must exert at least 65% of your maximal effort. When first starting, if you have been inactive, you must take it slowly. When walking, start with 10 minutes a day and try to increase it by five minutes a day, until you can walk vigorously for one hour, or about 25 miles a week.

Walk with a partner or your Battle Buddy, if you have a can; it makes the time go faster and allows some together time to talk and mutually support each other's efforts. As you become more capable, add some hand weights and pump your arms. You should be able to recite the Pledge of Allegiance while still breathing hard. Pulse rates are good guide lines and generally your maximum pulse rate should be around 220 minus your age in years.

Just taking increased "steps" as recorded by a personal pedometer has proven to be highly beneficial in motivating and sustaining increased walking in people who set goals of 10,000 steps a day. An inexpensive pedometer and even some phone apps. make it easy to record distance, and provides a record of your efforts, that can then be translated into excessive calories burned for inclusion in your dietary/work out dairy.

Find an exercise you like or at least don't despise. If being around others exercising inspires you, then join a class of exercise that you are pretty good at or can learn without risking injury. Spinning classes are popular and have a family sort of "we are all suffering together, but we will become an endorphin high family". Hiking is great, use walking sticks and carry water and a small pack up elevation to maximize benefit.

Swimming may truly be the fountain of youth. It conditions, very efficiently burns calories and does not produce joint trauma. Some of the best conditioned, optimal body weight seniors I have encountered in my medical practice are swimmers. They are a happy, high energy group who always look younger than their age.

Remember, any exercise is better than none. The benefits are immense and include not only weight loss acceleration and being better conditioned, but has been shown to decrease the incidence of "senile dementia" and to decrease depression. Without exercise, it is almost impossible to sustain a healthy body weight. There is no question that functional longevity directly correlates with life-long exercise. Become addicted, make it part of your life and reap the benefits.

CHAPTER 24:

SLEEP: A CRITICAL ELEMENT

Good sleep is critical to health. Prolonged sleep deprivation can cause complete breakdown of all of the systems of the body especially the brain and the immune system. If humans are deprived of sleep long enough, they will die.

Sleep is a mandatory anabolic state that allows rejuvenation, repair and growth of the brain, immune system, and skeletal muscle. It is essential for maintenance of memory, performing repetitive tasks, and problem solving. We now know that in the brain, repair and even growth of neurons and their connections, synapses, occurs during sleep.

Lack of healthy sleep has been linked directly to ASCVD, stroke, diabetes, hypertension and unhealthy weight gain. There is strong empirical evidence that inadequate sleep is a major risk factor for developing dementia. People that have inadequate sleep, irregular hours of sleeping, or who are chronically sleep deprived, die sooner and develop more disease that people with healthy sleep.

Recent studies have shown a link between lack of sleep and insulin resistance, the precursor to full blown diabetes. This effect is manifest in just two or three days of inadequate sleep. It is easy to extrapolate that chronic inadequate sleep is probably a major risk factor for developing diabetes.

When men are sleep deprived, their levels of ghrelin, the appetite stimulating hormone, go up much higher than usual. In women, it is not quite the same: their levels of leptin, the appetite "fullness" hormone go down, so they don't feel as satiated after eating. In males and females, lack of sleep stimulates over-eating and weight gain.

Children who get less than optimal sleep are heavier than those that do, and have a much greater incidence of diabetes and hypertension. The same has been demonstrated in teenagers. Babies, children and teenagers all require more sleep than adults, and if they get less than is optimal, there are potentially irreversible health consequences.

SLEEP APNEA

If you snore during the night, most likely someone who sleeps with you has enlightened you about the problem by now. Episodic snoring, getting louder, louder and louder, then stopping or pausing, without breathing for an apneic period, is probably sleep apnea. This disease is almost always associated with obesity. It is caused by a super fat tongue that drops down into the hypo pharynx, or back of the throat, during sleep, and blocks the air way, cutting off oxygen to the brain. The brain cannot live without oxygen, so it sends a message to wake up the afflicted victim. Such people are chronically exhausted; sleep on their feet, in the car, and at work for short periods, all day long. These victims are at massive risk for ASCVD, hypertension, stroke and diabetes.

If you suspect you might have sleep apnea, get your physician to order a sleep study and the diagnosis can be confirmed or ruled out. It is treated with a positive pressure breathing device, C-pap, worn at night, that prevents the blockage of the airway and hypoxia of the brain. Such treatment slows the progression of the associated lethal diseases. In many instances, losing the excessive weight eradicates the disease.

SLEEP STATE

Our individual internal circadian rhythm dictates our sleeping patterns. This physiologic internal clock is located somewhere in the deep brain, in an area called the hypothalamus. External clues like daylight and darkness send messages via the visual cortex of the brain and to the hypothalamus that regulate our individual internal clock. Our brain tells us when to sleep and when to be awake.

Each age has optimal hours of sleep a night. For most adults it is 7.5 to 9 hours a night. When preparing to sleep, the body temperature drops, the neuroactive substance, melatonin, and other sleep substances are released into the body causing us to become somnolent or sleepy. As we begin to sleep, our metabolic demands go down, our body temperature drops and we experience episodic temporary paralysis of our skeletal muscles.

There are very distinct stages of sleep that have been mapped by EEG, or brain waves. During a normal night of sleep, we will go through three stages of non-REM (rapid eye movement) sleep, and then into the dreaming sleep state, called REM sleep. We spend about 45% of our night's sleep in the non-REM state, stages I, II, and III. This non-REM sleep seems most important to the repair and rejuvenation of our brains, immune system and bodies. The non-REM sleep is important for maintaining declarative memory. Declarative memory is important for acquiring and maintaining facts, problem solving and general knowledge.

During a nightly 8 hour sleep, we cycle through the stages of non-REM sleep and then into REM sleep. This transition into deep reparative non-REM sleep then into REM sleep occurs approximately every 90 minutes and is marked by a short period of waking at the end of each cycle. On average, during an 8 hour night, most people have around 5 such cycles.

REM sleep is characterized by rapid movement of the eyes while they are closed, awake type EEG brain waves, and dreaming. We spend about 25% of our sleep time in REM sleep. REM sleep is the time that our muscles are temporarily paralyzed, and the parasympathetic nervous system is stimulated, frequently causing erections of the penis and clitoris. REM sleep is important for maintaining procedural memory. Procedural memory is important for completing repetitive acts, like tying shoes or playing tennis.

OPTIMAL SLEEP

THE BATTLE BUDDY DIET program requires optimal sleep. Experts agree that most adults need a solid 8 hours an night, give or take 1 hour, depending on the individual. It is simple, if you don't get optimal sleep, you will be unhealthy, at high risk for ASCVD, hypertension, obesity, diabetes and stroke. Lack of adequate sleep will make you want to eat more and be more inclined to eat the wrong, "lethal foods". A workaholic who claims to only "need 4 or 5 hours of sleep a night" is delusional and will eventually pay with loss of his/her health.

Make every effort to go to sleep at the same time every night. If it is the weekend and you are up later than usual, make a point of sleeping a full 8 hours before rising. If you work shift work, like I do, working late afternoons into the night, or even night shifts, make sure you establish a modified circadian rhythm that allows 8 hours of uninterrupted sleep during each 24 cycle. Try not to use sleep aid medications or alcohol to sleep: they all have side effects and interfere with the essential cycles of non-REM and REM sleep.

SLEEPING TIPS

Try to go to sleep at the same time every night. If you keep it regular, your body will expect it and be more ready to sleep. Try to have a one or two hour "wind down", get ready to sleep routine, or ritual that you repeat every night before sleeping.

Do not watch TV or use any video device, except an e-reader before bedtime. In fact, all electronic devices should be removed from the sleeping area. TV stimulates the brain, as do any lighted, LED type devices, even when your eyes are closed, and will inhibit the healthy transition between levels of sleep.

Use black-out drapes and use a sleeping mask to make your bedroom absolutely dark.

Avoid caffeine 8 hours before bedtime and limit the total amount to 2 cups of coffee a day.

Do not drink more than 2 oz. of alcohol before bedtime. Using alcohol to get to sleep, paradoxically prevents physiologic sleep, wakes you in the night, and only sedates you.

Exercise during the day, it makes you tired and decreases stress, allowing you to get to sleep easier.

Keep a pad and pen in the bedside table to write down those, "I've got to remember to do so-and-so, tomorrow" thoughts that will keep you awake with anxiety. Once you write them down, they are there and you won't forget, and can remove them from you brain.

If your sleeping partner snores, get ear plugs and a white noise machine. Turn the machine up to block out the snoring. Such a machine saved my marriage.

Avoid doing stressful things before bedtime. Return that call to your bipolar sister tomorrow. Don't look at your projected quarterly taxes right before bed. Watch a mindless TV show, there are many available, or read a good book.

Use that phone answering machine, and turn off the phones in your bedroom. Unless you are a surgeon on call, or have teenagers out of the house driving, most calls can wait until the morning.

Reading to fall asleep works, because it is brain active, unlike TV, and makes your brain tired.

Do not eat a large meal right before retiring, a snack is fine.

Put a glass of water by the bedside. Do not drink excessive fluids in the hours before bedtime.

Get the dog or cat a pet bed, to put at the foot of your bed. Don't let them sleep in the bed with you; they will interrupt your 90 minute sleep cycles by waking you up.

Keep the bedroom cool to cold, and use comfortable warm covers. Crack a bedroom window.

Invest in a top of the line mattress; it is a good investment.

BIOGRAPHY: COL R.D. SLAY, M.D.

Colonel (RET) Robert Slay M.D. USA is a practicing Emergency physician, who is board-certified in Internal Medicine and Emergency Medicine. He is a graduate of the Virginia Military Institute and the Medical College of Virginia. He served in the U. S. Army as an emergency physician for twenty two years. He was a member of the elite Delta Force, and retired as a Colonel.

Dr. Slay has contributed to several textbooks in Emergency Medicine, has been elected a Fellow of the American College of Emergency Medicine, and the American Academy of Emergency Medicine, and currently serves as an oral examiner for the American Board of Emergency Medicine. Dr. Slay has extensively researched nutrition and life-style, aided and abetted by his wife, and "Battle Buddy", Gayne Brenneman, M.D.

Dr. Slay has become frustrated in his Emergency Medicine practice taking care of the end stage of diseases brought on by obesity, lethal foods and unhealthy life-style. The tsunami of sick baby boomers flooding the ER with self-induced diseases is only increasing. Taking care of them "feels like trying to put a band aid on a bleeding artery: "Too little, too late"

After researching the medical literature, Dr. Slay and his wife realized they were at risk for the same obesity linked diseases, because they had truncal obesity and ate the wrong foods. They developed their own program of healthy nutrition, and life-style, THE BATTLE BUDDY DIET, and applied it to their own lives and became remarkably healthier and happier in just 4 weeks.

Their physician colleagues, woefully ignorant about nutrition and life-style, wanted to know, "How did you do it?" Dr. Slay decided to write the book, THE BATTLE BUDDY DIET, to educate physicians and patients on how to save their own lives and their children's. He and his wife are convinced that couples can do it together as "Battle Buddies" relying on mutual commitment and support, in only 4 weeks.

Dr. Slay has written scripts for and acted in the reality based medical television show, "Untold Stories of the ER" for six episodes. He performs Emergency Room stand-up comedy as a hobby.

Please feel free to share your experience and story with us through our web site: battlebuddydiet.com.

PREEFACE

DOCTORS' DIET FOR DOCTORS

RECLAIM YOUR LIFE

THE REAL TRUTH FROM A DOCTOR COUPLE WHO HAVE DONE IT.

YOUR GUIDE TO A LIFE SAVING, LIFE-STYLE CHANGE, BY A HUSBAND AND WIFE PHYSICIAN COUPLE.

HOW BODY FAT IS A DEATH SENTENCE, WILL SHORTEN YOUR LIFE, AND LEAD TO DISABILITY WITH AGING

THE TWELVE LETHAL FOODS THAT YOU SHOULD NEVER EAT AGAIN

IF YOU HAVE HAD ENOUGH, AND WANT TO TAKE CONTROL OF YOUR BODY FAT, AND WHAT YOU EAT, AND ARE WILLING TO COMMITT TO A REAL LIFE-STYLE CHANGE, WITH DIET, EXERCISE AND WEIGHT LIFTING. THIS IS HOW TO DO IT SAFELY, SURELY, AND WITH LASTING RESULTS.

IDEAL BODY WEIGHT WILL MAKE YOU LOOK YOUR BEST RIGHT NOW, SLOW AGING, GIVE YOU MORE ENERGY, TURBO-CHARGE YOUR SEX LIFE, AND PREVENT THE OBESITY RELATED DISEASES WHICH ALL LEAD TO DISABILITY, AND LIFE LONG DEPENDENCY ON MEDICINES, DOCTORS AND HOSPITALS.

THIS IS HOW A DOCTOR COUPLE DID IT, BASED ON A CAREFUL REVIEW OF THE REAL SCIENTIFIC FACTS, SUPPORTED BY CREDIBLE, WELL DONE STUDIES, ENDORSED BY THE WHO, CDC, NIH, NIA, AND UNIVERSITY/ CURRENT AND ON-GOING ACADEMIC STUDIES, CONCERNING DIET, AGING, OBESITY AND RISK FACTORS FOR MULTIPLE DISEASES.

THIS MATERIAL IS FACTUAL, THE REAL TRUTH, NOT INFLUNENCED BY ANY LOBBY, FOOD PRODUCERS, OR ELIXIR SALESMEN.

Made in the USA
San Bernardino, CA
03 December 2013